YOUR
CARB
Diary

11673176

YOUR CARB *Diary*

Shelagh Ryan Masline

A Lynn Sonberg Book

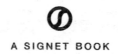

A SIGNET BOOK

SIGNET
Published by New American Library, a division of
Penguin Group (USA) Inc., 375 Hudson Street, New York, New York 10014, U.S.A.
Penguin Books Ltd, 80 Strand, London WC2R 0RL, England
Penguin Books Australia Ltd, 250 Camberwell Road,
Camberwell, Victoria 3124, Australia
Penguin Books Canada Ltd, 10 Alcorn Avenue, Toronto, Ontario, Canada M4V 3B2
Penguin Books (N.Z.) Ltd, Cnr Rosedale and Airborne Roads,
Albany, Auckland 1310, New Zealand

Penguin Books Ltd, Registered Offices: 80 Strand, London WC2R 0RL, England

First published by Signet, an imprint of New American Library, a division of Penguin
Group (USA) Inc.

First Printing, March 2004
10   9   8   7   6   5   4   3

Copyright © Lynn Sonberg, 2004
All rights reserved

Ⓢ REGISTERED TRADEMARK—MARCA REGISTRADA

Printed in the United States of America

Without limiting the rights under copyright reserved above, no part of this publica-
tion may be reproduced, stored in or introduced into a retrieval system, or trans-
mitted, in any form, or by any means (electronic, mechanical, photocopying,
recording, or otherwise), without the prior written permission of both the copyright
owner and the above publisher of this book.

PUBLISHER'S NOTE
Every effort as been made to ensure that the information contained in this book is
complete and accurate. However, neither the publisher nor the author is engaged
in rendering professional advice or services to the individual reader. The ideas, pro-
cedures, and suggestions contained in this book are not intended as a substitute
for consulting with your physician. All matters regarding your health require medical
supervision. Neither the author nor the publisher shall be liable or responsible for any
loss or damage allegedly arising from any information or suggestion in this book.

BOOKS ARE AVAILABLE AT QUANTITY DISCOUNTS WHEN USED TO PRO-
MOTE PRODUCTS OR SERVICES. FOR INFORMATION PLEASE WRITE TO
PREMIUM MARKETING DIVISION, PENGUIN GROUP (USA) INC., 375 HUDSON
STREET, NEW YORK, NEW YORK 10014.

The scanning, uploading and distribution of this book via the Internet or via any
other means without the permission of the publisher is illegal and punishable by
law. Please purchase only authorized electronic editions, and do not participate in
or encourage electronic piracy of copyrighted materials. Your support of the author's
rights is appreciated.

To my best helper, Caitlin

ACKNOWLEDGMENTS

This book was a team project. Many thanks to computer whiz Caitlin Ryan Masline for her invaluable assistance with all things graphic or chartlike, and for her helpful dietary suggestions from Gail Shu's ninth grade biology class. Thanks too to Lynn Sonberg for thinking of me for this project and for her remarkably rapid as well as perceptive editing and overall input.

ACKNOWLEDGMENTS

INTRODUCTION

HOW TO USE *YOUR CARB DIARY*

Whether you're counting carbs to shed pounds, to maintain a healthy weight, or simply to enhance your health overall, a diary is an invaluable tool to help you meet your goals. In one slim volume, *Your Carb Diary* has everything you need to begin your healthy new low-carb lifestyle:

- The facts on what low-carb diets are, how they work, and how to follow them; the positive impact a low-carb lifestyle will have on your health; and a quick peek at a few of the most popular low-carb diets, including Atkins and South Beach.
- A twenty-six-week diary, in which you can keep track of exactly what you eat and drink each day; your daily exercise ("Let's get physical"); and your thoughts and feelings about the obstacles you face and the progress you make ("How am I doing?").
- A carb counter, where you can quickly and easily look up the carbs, fiber, net carbs, and calories of 300 common foods.

The Problem: Too Much Sugar and White Flour

We've come a long way from the all-fats-are-bad and it's-okay-to-eat-all-the-low-fat-cookies-you-want mentality. Today we know the truth: Sure, food manufacturers took the fat out of cookies, but to compensate for the loss in flavor, they loaded up on sweeteners like carb-heavy sugar and high-fructose corn syrup!

The famous Food Guide Pyramid created by the U.S. Department of Agriculture (USDA) in 1992 is an object lesson in how *not* to eat: It makes no distinction between refined carbs and whole carbs. All bread, cereal, rice, and pasta are lumped together at the bottom of the pyramid, and we were told to eat 6 to 11 servings of them every day. We did, and as a society, we got fat!

Along with the rest of the medical powers that be, the USDA created the impression that all carbs are good and all fats are bad. Now, at the department of nutrition at the Harvard School of Public Health, Dr. Walter Willett has designed a better alternative: a food pyramid that places whole-grain foods near the base (to be eaten most frequently) and white rice, white bread, potatoes, pasta, and sweets at the top of the pyramid (to be consumed sparingly). This is more like it.

You've probably read about the twin epidemics of obesity and diabetes in this country. Many experts believe that empty carbs such as sugar and white flour are the reason for these problems, and watching carbs is the solution.

The Solution: Count Carbs

The low-fat diet has given way to the low-carb diet, and signs of the low-carb revolution are everywhere around us. Restaurants are joining in, listing carbohydrate values on their menus, while food manufacturers are busily rolling out new low-carb or carb-free product lines. And now when you go out to eat or to shop for your weekly groceries, you have your own portable carb detection kit: *Your Carb Diary*. Just tuck it into your pocket or handbag.

So how does the low-carb diet work? When you eat a piece of white bread or a bag of corn chips, glucose (blood sugar) rushes into your bloodstream. In response, your body produces insulin to allow glucose to enter the body's cells for energy. If there is more glucose than the body's cells need, the excess is temporarily stored as glycogen.

Once there is enough glycogen in storage, insulin prompts the liver to convert excess glucose into body fat.

In a nutshell? The more carbs you eat, the more insulin you produce, the more excess body fat you store. When you reduce your carbohydrate intake, you'll shed excess pounds. It's as simple as that.

To plan dietary strategies for your first official week of low-carb living, turn directly to the carb counter on page 209. Or plunge right in and get started on your diary, which begins on page 1. But first, read on to learn in greater detail about carbs and how they affect your health.

Before You Begin Counting Carbs

Should I see my physician before I start a low-carb diet plan?
Absolutely. A complete medical checkup is a must before starting any new diet plan. This is especially important if you have a preexisting condition such as diabetes, kidney disease, or cardiovascular problems. Your doctor may check your cholesterol levels, triglycerides (blood fats), glucose level, insulin level, and thyroid function.

Will following a low-carb diet affect my prescriptions?
This is a question that you must ask your doctor. In some cases, a low-carb, high-protein diet *will* have an impact on your need for prescription medications. For example, low-carb diets are naturally diuretic and if you are taking a diuretic, your dosage may need to be adjusted downward. Diabetics may have to adjust their dosage of insulin, and weight loss may lead to a reduction in blood pressure medication.

What other questions should I ask my doctor?

Inform your physician if you're planning to go super low-carb (in the range of 20 net carbs daily). If so, ask whether ketosis—a state in which the body burns fat because no carbohydrates are readily available—presents any health concerns for you. (Read more about ketosis on page xxvi.)

Should I take a daily multivitamin and mineral supplement?

This is generally a good idea for everyone, especially when embarking on a new diet.

Why count carbs?

Some people monitor carb intake for weight loss, while others want to maintain a healthy weight and reduce the amount of empty carbohydrates such as white flour and sugar in their diets. The fact is, weight loss and overall health are closely connected. If you are overweight, even a modest weight loss pays off in health benefits. For example, losing just a few pounds cuts the risk of heart disease.

What are net carbs?

These are the carbs that you need to keep close track of in your new low-carb lifestyle. Certain carbs—namely fiber, glycerine, and sugar alcohols—do not impact blood sugar and are not counted as net carbs. Net carbohydrates are those that can be digested by your body and have a direct impact on blood sugar. To learn the number of net carbs in a food, refer to your carb counter or check the label. If net carbs are not listed individually in the label, simply subtract fiber grams from total carbohydrates. That's your net carb number.

Why is the impact on blood sugar so important?
Fiber-rich whole grains are broken down slowly in the digestive system. In contrast, refined carbs and simple sugars rush into the bloodstream as glucose. If glucose is not quickly used to fuel activity, the body produces insulin to take it out of circulation and convert it into fat.

What is the daily carb quota?
This is how many carbs you want to limit yourself to each day. At the beginning of each week, write this number down in *Your Carb Diary*.

How do I know what my daily carb quota is?
For weight loss, the average daily carb quota is between 40 and 60 net grams. Some people—mainly men—manage to lose weight while consuming as much as 100 net carbs daily.

  If you follow the Atkins plan, in the early weeks you limit yourself to a very low 20 net carbs daily. Then you gradually increase your daily net carb intake by 5 grams weekly, until you stop losing weight. Subtract 5 and that's your daily carb quota—the maximum number of carbs you can consume and still lose weight.

What can I eat at a daily carb quota of 20 net grams?
To give you an idea of what 20 net carb grams means, a soda, a plain bagel, a cup of cereal, and a bag of potato chips each contains more than 20 net carb grams! So what carbs *can* you eat? Three cups of salad greens with low-carb dressing, or 2 cups of salad and 1 cup of a nonstarchy vegetable such as broccoli or asparagus.

But won't that leave me uncomfortably hungry?
No, because you're only counting carbs—not protein or fat. With your salad or veggies, you can have steak, chicken, pork chops, salmon, tuna, tofu, eggs, or other foods high in protein and/or healthy fats (such as olive oil). Cheese is also allowed in limited quantities. This is one of the great benefits of the low-carb lifestyle: It doesn't leave you feeling deprived, as low-fat diets typically do!

Does this mean I can eat unlimited quantities of bacon and well-marbled steak at every meal?!
No. In fact, you've uncovered one of the great misconceptions about low-carb diets. Most low-carb diet plans recommend *moderate portions* of *high-quality* proteins and *healthy* fats. For example, a 6-ounce portion of grilled salmon or tuna contains no carbohydrates and is moreover a rich source of heart-healthy omega-3 fatty acids.

Are there any fish or meats that should be avoided?
You should generally steer clear of fish or meat products (such as bacon) that are cured with nitrates, which are known carcinogens. Other meats to watch out for are processed cold cuts (such as salami, bologna, and ham) that may contain sugar or other fillers that add carbs. Ditto for meat loaf, fish sticks, and any other breaded products.

Does it matter how food is prepared?
Yes. In addition to breading, beware of sauces, marinades, and gravies. These are common sources of hidden carbohydrates and can easily sabotage a low-carb weight loss plan. As far as cooking techniques go, grilling, baking, poaching, and steaming are always healthier choices than frying.

How do I go about counting net carbs?

When you use *Your Carb Diary*, it's very easy. Just turn to the counter on page 209 and look up whatever food you are eating. Foods are grouped under categories, such as Vegetables, Poultry, or Baked Goods and Snacks.

Every day, record the net carbs that you consume at each meal and snack. Don't forget to count carbs in beverages as well as foods! And at the top of each diary entry, note the total number of net carbs you consumed that day.

What types of carbs should I avoid?

Avoid the fluffy white carbs, such as white flour, white rice, white sugar, and potatoes. Some dieters even refer to white bread as the White Devil! In general, it's important to steer clear of processed foods, which are packed with empty, nutrient-poor carbs and calories. The problem has gone way beyond conventional junk foods like chips, candy, and cookies. Even most processed cereals—once thought to be a great source of nutrition—are made with refined grains that have been leached of nutritional value. Not to mention the sugar content of breakfast cereals whose names sound more like those of candy bars! Sodas and sports drinks are also loaded with sugar. Make a point to check the labels and refer to your carb counter.

What are examples of good carbs?

There are many healthy carbs that you can and should include in your diet. These include asparagus, avocados, broccoli, cauliflower, onion, peppers, spinach, squash, tomatoes, blueberries, raspberries, strawberries, cantaloupe, honeydew, kiwi, rhubarb, sunflower seeds, macadamia nuts, walnuts, almonds, and pecans. Because berries are high in fiber and low in carbs, they're a low-carb favorite.

Nutrient-rich as they are, it's better to avoid whole grains and legumes in your initial weight loss period. As time goes on and you get closer to your ideal weight, you can gradually reincorporate more nutritious beans, whole-grain breads, brown rice, and bulgur and other grains into your diet.

The key is to watch your net carb count, avoid junk foods and other empty carbs, and eat a variety of healthy foods in moderation.

How do I use the carb counter?

Next to each item in the counter, you will see four categories:

- *Carbs:* The total number of carbs in a food, including fiber.
- *Fiber:* The indigestible parts of plant cells. Unlike other carbohydrates, fiber doesn't convert to glucose and raise your blood sugar. The higher the fiber number, the better it is for your health.
- *Net carbs:* The carbohydrates that can be digested by your body and have a direct impact on blood sugar. When it comes to this number, the lower the better. Record your daily consumption of net carbs in your diary.
- *Calories:* A measurement of energy provided by food. Carbohydrates and fats are the body's main sources of energy, and excess calories are stored as body fat. Although carbs are the key to weight loss, many dieters still find it helpful to keep an eye on calorie counts.

Why is it necessary to drink so much water on a low-carb diet?

Water flushes the toxins from your body, keeps you hydrated, and helps prevent constipation. Every day, drink at least eight 8-ounce glasses of tap water, filtered water, spring water, or mineral water—and remember to keep track of your intake in *Your Carb Diary*. Other beverages, such as club soda or herbal teas, are also fine. Of course, avoid sugary sodas and sports drinks (which are high in carbohydrates), and drink only moderate amounts of coffee and tea (which are diuretics). Use a sugar substitute such as sucralose (marketed as Splenda) to sweeten tea, coffee, or lemonade.

In week one, I record my current and my target weight and clothing size. But why measure my waist?
Many people think a slender waist is more attractive and make it part of their weight loss goal. But even if you're not seriously overweight, extra inches around your waist are unhealthy. It's important to know your waist circumference because so-called apple shaped bodies are associated with a higher risk of heart disease, high blood pressure, high cholesterol, and diabetes. Women with a waist circumference of 35 inches or more and men with a waist circumference of 40 inches or more are at greater disease risk. But the good news is that counting your carbs can help you whittle down that waist.

Why is exercise so important?
Exercise is a key component of any weight loss plan. In fact, even if you're going low-carb to maintain a healthy weight or to cut out the junk foods, it's vital to stay active and, ideally, work out on a regular basis. Keep in mind that you don't have to morph into a gym rat or marathon runner. If you've been inactive, even modest amounts of exercise are beneficial. For example, start out with a brisk walk for 20 to 30 minutes three to four times a week. After even just a week or two, you'll be amazed at how much stronger and more energetic you feel.

I'm always hungry on low-fat diets. Will I experience food cravings on a low-carb plan?

You shouldn't. As I mentioned earlier, a signature benefit of low-carb diets is that the protein and fat you eat leave you feeling satisfied rather than hungry. To have more control over your diet and to keep blood sugar on an even keel, eat a number of small, regular meals. Also, space your carb intake evenly throughout the day and avoid high-carb snacking.

Of course, cravings *can* develop if you cheat! For example, if you have a high-carb snack such as a bag of cookies or chips, you will experience an immediate surge in blood sugar, followed by a later drop in energy that leaves you craving something sweet.

If you're not cheating and you still have consistent problems with cravings, cut back on your daily carb quota and increase your consumption of protein and fat.

What do I do if I get discouraged and want to quit?

Here's where your diary really comes in handy! Use your own words to motivate yourself. Relive the challenges you've successfully faced—resolutely walking by the neighborhood bakery without going in, forgoing the candy and other snack machines that beckon to you siren-like at the office. Sure, you may slip a few times—who doesn't? But that doesn't mean you should give up. Leaf back through the pages of *Your Carb Diary* to see how far you've already come!

ALL ABOUT CARBS: A PRIMER

You've already read enough to help you get started on your lower carb eating plan, but if you want a deeper understanding of how and why carbs are the key to losing weight—and staying healthy—read on!

Let's get down to the nitty gritty. Why all the fuss about carbs?

While not everybody agrees, there is a growing body of evidence suggesting that the problem with the typical American diet has more to do with excess carbohydrates than fat. Eating too many carbohydrates like sugar and white flour:

- Raises insulin levels, which increases the risk of health problems such as diabetes.
- Raises the level of fats in our blood called triglycerides, which increases the risk of cardiovascular disease.
- Makes us fat, because the more carbs you eat, the more insulin you produce, the more fat you store. Being overweight leads to diabetes and heart disease, and raises our risk factors for a variety of other health problems, including cancer.

Why don't low-fat diets work?

It turns out that the public health authorities' previous take on fat was way off target. Losing weight and enhancing health is not, after all, just about counting and avoiding grams of fat. In fact, some fats (such as those in monounsaturated olive oil and in cold water fish such as salmon) are not only beneficial, they are necessary to our health. And the diet we were encouraged to embrace as an alternative—loading up on the pasta and low-fat sweets—has been a major contributor to the current epidemic of obesity in this country.

So what fats are bad for you?

The saturated fat in beef, pork, and milk products and the trans fats in processed products and deep-fried fast foods are major contributors to obesity and heart disease. Created by adding hydrogen to vegetable oil (which solidifies it and increases shelf life), trans fats were first manufactured in the 1980s as an alternative to unhealthy saturated fats. Today, thousands of foods are packed with trans-fatty acids, from margarine and shortening to French fries and chicken nuggets. Ironically, however, it turns out that trans fats are even *worse* for us than saturated fats. Not only do they raise "bad" LDL cholesterol levels and triglycerides, these fats also lower "good" HDL cholesterol.

How do I know if a food contains trans-fatty acids? Are they listed on the label?
The U.S. Food and Drug Administration (FDA) recently announced that all food processors must list trans-fatty acid content on their labels by 2006. In the meantime, your tip-off on food labels is "partially hydrogenated vegetable oil"—the code name for trans fats! Foods such as crackers, cookies, white bread, and doughnuts typically contain not only trans fats but also white flour and added sweeteners—meaning that they have high carbs, low fiber, and deadly fats. A dangerous combination!

And what fats are good for you?
Unlike trans-fatty acids and saturated fats, essential fatty acids are good for our health and protect against heart disease. Good sources of healthy fats include avocados, fatty fish (salmon, sea bass, trout, etc.), nuts, seeds, natural peanut butter, and a variety of oils, especially canola, olive, sesame, and flaxseed.

So cutting back on fat and bulking up on carbs is not the answer?
No! The problem is that many of the low- and no-fat products lining supermarket shelves are packed with empty carbs like sugar and corn syrup to compensate for the loss in taste when fat is removed. Remember those low-fat

cookies I mentioned earlier? You probably assumed—in fact, food manufacturers *encouraged* you to assume—that because they contained little fat, you could eat as many as you wanted without gaining weight. But eat too many calories, no matter where they come from (protein, carbohydrate, or fat), and you will gain weight. If you eat a box of low-fat cookies, the calories are going to add up . . . and any calories consumed beyond what your body burns are stored as body fat.

How does eating carbs contribute to obesity and related health problems?

More than two decades of low-fat recommendations from health authorities from the surgeon general on down have had no impact on the level of heart disease in this country and have coincided with a steep increase in obesity and diabetes. Low-carb advocates believe that this is no coincidence. Basically, we followed the medical establishment's advice to eat more fat-free carbohydrates. This made us hungrier, fatter, and more susceptible to diabetes and heart disease.

How common is obesity? And how does being overweight affect your health?

According to the latest government figures, about two out of three Americans are overweight or obese. These excess pounds are linked to a host of health problems, including high blood pressure, heart disease, stroke, diabetes, gallstones, arthritis, cancer, and more. About 300,000 deaths each year are linked to obesity.

Exactly what are carbohydrates anyway?

Carbohydrates, which include sugars, fibers, and starches, are the body's main source of energy. These compounds occur in most foods, including bread, pasta, potatoes, bananas, cookies, pies, lentils, couscous, soft drinks, and milk. Of course, different types of carbohydrates are present in different foods.

Are all carbs bad for you?

Of course not. As with that of dietary fat, the role of carbohydrates cannot be boiled down to a simplistic "They're good for you" or "They're bad for you." The effect of these nutrients on our health is complex, and you need to look not only at the amount of carbohydrates you eat, but the type. The sugar and white flour in junk foods provide only empty calories, but lots of carbohydrates—such as fiber-rich fresh vegetables and whole, unrefined grains—can play important roles in a healthy diet. Scientists classify carbohydrates as simple or complex. Simple carbohydrates include the single and double sugars. Complex carbs consist of glycogen, starch, and fiber.

How are sugars identified on food labels?

It's important to read labels carefully, because food manufacturers identify sugar under many different names. Also check portion sizes, which may be smaller than you realize. Terms for sugar include:

- brown sugar
- corn sweetener
- corn syrup
- dextrose
- fructose
- fruit juice concentrate
- glucose
- high-fructose corn syrup
- honey
- lactose
- malt or malt syrup
- maltose
- molasses
- raw sugar
- sucrose

What happens in the body when you consume sugar?
Simple sugars quickly flood the bloodstream. If that glucose is not used immediately as fuel, insulin prompts the liver to store excess glucose in a temporary form known as glycogen. This can be tapped as necessary as a quick source of energy. Once the body has stored a sufficient amount of glycogen, insulin again acts, this time causing the liver to convert any remaining glucose to body fat for more permanent storage.

What is starch?
This is the form in which plants—such as wheat, corn, rice, and potatoes—store unused glucose.

What is fiber?
Fiber, which is found in every plant we eat, is a nondigestible carbohydrate. This means that it is not absorbed into the bloodstream, so it has no direct impact on insulin. The higher the fiber content of a carbohydrate, the slower its rate of absorption into the bloodstream.

What does fiber do in the body?
It performs a number of valuable functions. Fiber:
- Eases constipation
- Decreases the risk of hemorrhoids and irritable bowel syndrome
- Decreases appetite
- Slows glucose absorption

What happens in the body when you consume fiber?
Fiber is absorbed differently from all other carbohydrates, whether simple or complex. Because it actually slows the rate of glucose absorption—while other carbs speed it up—fiber is not included in your daily net carb count.

How are low-carb diets superior to low-fat diets?

With the notable exception of fiber-rich vegetables and whole grains, the vast majority of carbs consumed by Americans are junk foods loaded with sugar and refined flour. Every day we consume about 300 carb grams . . . far more than we can use as fuel. In the body, these carbs are rapidly converted into glucose; in response, the pancreas pumps out insulin to rush glucose into cells for use as energy; and whatever glucose is not used as fuel is stored as fat.

Low-carb diets address the true culprits in weight gain: carbohydrates and insulin. With obesity and diabetes on the rise, it's clear that the old approach—limiting calories and fat—just didn't do the trick. Over time, the body gets used to—some even say addicted to—carbohydrates. You may also become gradually resistant to using insulin efficiently. Replacing carbs with healthy proteins and fats will leave you feeling satisfied instead of deprived and hungry, empower you to reduce your reliance on carbs, and help you switch from burning carbs to burning fat.

What is insulin?

Insulin is a hormone produced by the pancreas that helps your body use sugar in the food you eat as fuel. It enables glucose to enter cells.

What is insulin resistance?

In some people—especially those who are already overweight—tissues in the body stop responding to insulin. When cells become resistant to insulin's action, the pancreas pumps out even more insulin in an attempt to force sugar into the cells.

How is insulin resistance different from diabetes?
In insulin resistance, your blood sugar level is not quite high enough to constitute diabetes, but it is higher than normal. Each year about 5 percent of people with insulin resistance go on to develop type 2 diabetes. A recent study also showed insulin resistance to be a significant risk factor for heart attacks.

How is being overweight related to insulin resistance and type 2 diabetes?
When you're overweight, you're more likely to develop type 2 diabetes, a disorder characterized by insulin resistance that interferes with the body's ability to use glucose. On the other hand, you may be overweight because you're insulin resistant, and insulin resistance makes it difficult to lose weight. By cutting carbs, you can break your way out of this vicious cycle of excess insulin and excess pounds. When you have fewer carbs to process, your body produces less insulin. Instead, you begin to burn fat and shed excess pounds. In some diabetics, this may even mean that you can control your disorder through diet and exercise and no longer need to use glucose-lowering drugs.

How does insulin resistance increase the risk of heart attacks?
Excess insulin directly damages coronary arteries. It also triggers a set of metabolic abnormalities that contributes to the development of artery-clogging plaque and blood clots. This dangerous syndrome is known as syndrome X.

What are the characteristics of syndrome X?
- High levels of triglycerides, the body's primary fat storage particles
- Low levels of "good" HDL cholesterol

- Excess fibrinogen, a substance that promotes blood clots
- Excess plasminogen activator inhibitor-1 (PAI-1), a substance that slows clot breakdown

Are there any other health problems associated with insulin resistance and syndrome X?

Many people with syndrome X also have high blood pressure. They're also more likely to have polycystic ovary syndrome, a fatty liver, and certain types of cancer.

What can I do to reverse insulin resistance?

Control carbohydrate intake! To moderate or even reverse insulin resistance, limit your intake of refined carbohydrates such as white flour and sugar that raise blood sugar and triglyceride levels. Increase your intake of protein, which doesn't require your body to produce so much insulin because there is no need to cope with sudden surges of blood sugar.

What is ketosis?

Ketosis is an important part of the early weeks of Atkins and some other low-carb plans. It works like this: When carbohydrates are *extremely* limited in the diet, insulin falls very low, and the body begins to burn stored fat. In effect, you have switched your body from a glucose metabolism to a fat metabolism, because you are burning your body fat for energy instead of storing it.

Why is ketosis controversial?

Burning fats without carbohydrates creates byproducts called ketones that begin to accumulate in the bloodstream. Ketones suppress appetite, but may also cause nausea and fatigue. Your kidneys remove ketones in the bloodstream and eliminate them in urine.

Ketosis is a state that normally occurs during fasting and starvation. According to Atkins, ketosis is an effective way to jump-start weight loss. Some critics claim that it is dangerous. But this has never been proven, and many low-carb advocates believe that critics are confusing ketosis with ketoacidosis—a potentially fatal condition in diabetics.

What is the glycemic index?
This is another way of looking at carbohydrates. Basically, the glycemic index measures how quickly blood sugar rises after you eat foods that contain carbohydrates. Refined carbs like white bread, pasta, crackers, and cornflakes cause a very rapid rise in blood sugar, so they are assigned a high glycemic index. The idea is to consume low-glycemic-index foods, which are absorbed slowly. According to this thinking, you can eat a wider range of carbs as long as they are fairly low on the glycemic scale, including apricots, cherries, grapefruit, tomatoes, lentils, black beans, chickpeas, soy beans, oatmeal, brown rice, wheat bran, oat bran, whole-grain breads, bulgur, barley, whole-grain breakfast cereals, and couscous.

Can you talk about a few of the popular low-carb diet plans?
From the once controversial Atkins plan to the wildly popular South Beach diet, today there is a plethora of low-carb, high-protein diet plans developed in response to increasing interest in low carbs. All advise limiting carbohydrates rather than fat in the diet.

What about Atkins?

Atkins is the powerhouse of all the low-carb diet plans. Way back in 1972, Dr. Robert C. Atkins was the first to postulate that carbs—not fat—were the problem behind widespread weight gain. At that time, Dr. Atkins was made a virtual pariah by the medical establishment for his unorthodox views. But the years have borne out his theory: When carbs are not available, the body burns fat for energy.

The Atkins plan is good for short-term weight loss, but no study has thus far verified sustained long-term weight loss. The earliest weeks are the toughest on this low-carb plan, when dieters are advised to limit themselves to a sparse 20 daily net carbs—the equivalent of three cups of salad with low-carb dressing. The good part is that since dieters are allowed higher amounts of fat, they feel satisfied, not deprived as in traditional diets.

What is the South Beach diet?

The South Beach diet is not strictly low-fat or low-carb. Instead, its creator, cardiologist Dr. Arthur Agatston, emphasizes the right carbs and right fats. South Beach retains the best parts of Atkins, such as the emphasis on healthy proteins, while not totally excluding carbs. Dr. Agatston encourages including plenty of fruits, vegetables, whole grains, nuts, and healthy oils in your diet. Still, by making the right choices, he says, you can lose as many as 8 to 13 pounds in the first two weeks.

How about the Zone?

Like the top athletes that author Dr. Barry Sears has worked with over the years, you have the goal on this diet to reach and spend as much time as possible in the Zone. To accomplish this, your daily food intake should consist of 30 percent protein, 30 percent fat, and 40 percent carbohydrates. The theory goes that reaching the Zone, which requires precise control of the protein-to-carbohydrate ratio, stimulates the optimum production of insulin. This encourages weight loss and other health benefits, such as enhanced mental productivity and disease prevention. The Zone emphasizes proteins that are low in saturated fat. Unlike Atkins, it does not involve ketosis.

What is the Sugar Busters! diet?

According to H. Leighton Steward and his coauthors, the problem is sugar . . . and low-fat food is full of sugar. Sugar causes the production of insulin, which can keep you from losing weight no matter how much you diet and exercise. *Sugar Busters!* encourages you to reduce your daily consumption of sugar and steers you away from insulin-stimulating foods such as pasta, potatoes, white bread, white rice, carrots, and corn. To measure how quickly blood sugar rises after eating various carbs, *Sugar Busters!* utilizes the glycemic index. Tips include avoiding food combinations that add pounds (such as fruit with meat) and choosing appropriate times of day to eat foods (for instance, do not eat a large meal shortly before going to bed).

YOUR
CARB
Diary

WEEK ONE

Congratulations! You're about to take your first step on the road to a fitter and healthier, slimmer and trimmer, more energetic new you.

Use this twenty-six-week diary to record your physical and emotional progress. Each day, write down what you eat, your net carb intake, how many glasses of water you drink (remember that your goal is eight 8-ounce glasses), how much you've exercised, and your thoughts and feelings about the challenges you face and the goals you achieve. To get started, record your vital starting stats (and target stats) below.

Next, decide how many net carbs you will be consuming each day this week. To achieve weight loss, you should have an average daily carb quota of between 40 and 60 net grams. Some people prefer to jumpstart their diets by limiting themselves to just 20 grams a day for the first two weeks, while others can lose weight consuming as many as 100 net carbs daily. Of course, as discussed in the introduction, always check with your doctor before making any major changes in your diet.

Weight: _____

Target Weight: _____

Clothing Size: _____

Target Clothing Size: _____

Waist Measurement: _____

Target Waist Measurement: _____

Daily Carb Quota: _____

SUNDAY

Date: _____

Total Daily Net Carb Intake: _____

BREAKFAST:

Net Carbs: _____

LUNCH:

Net Carbs: _____

DINNER:

Net Carbs: _____

SNACKS:
   Morning:
   Afternoon:
   Evening:

Net Carbs: _____

Glasses of Water: _____

Let's Get Physical: _____
_____
_____
_____

How Am I Doing?: _____
_____
_____
_____

MONDAY

Date: _____

Total Daily Net Carb Intake: _____

BREAKFAST:

Net Carbs: _____

LUNCH:

Net Carbs: _____

DINNER:

Net Carbs: _____

SNACKS:
  Morning:
  Afternoon:
  Evening:

Net Carbs: _____

Glasses of Water: _____

Let's Get Physical: _____

_____

_____

_____

How Am I Doing?: _____

_____

_____

_____

TUESDAY

Date: _____

Total Daily Net Carb Intake: _____

BREAKFAST:

Net Carbs: _____

LUNCH:

Net Carbs: _____

DINNER:

Net Carbs: _____

SNACKS:
Morning:
Afternoon:
Evening:

Net Carbs: _____

Glasses of Water: _____

Let's Get Physical: _____
_____
_____
_____

How Am I Doing?: _____
_____
_____
_____

WEDNESDAY

Date: _____

Total Daily Net Carb Intake: _____

BREAKFAST:

Net Carbs: _____

LUNCH:

Net Carbs: _____

DINNER:

Net Carbs: _____

SNACKS:
   Morning:
   Afternoon:
   Evening:

Net Carbs: _____

Glasses of Water: _____

Let's Get Physical: _____
_____
_____
_____

How Am I Doing?: _____
_____
_____
_____

THURSDAY

Date: _____

Total Daily Net Carb Intake: _____

BREAKFAST:

Net Carbs: _____

LUNCH:

Net Carbs: _____

DINNER:

Net Carbs: _____

SNACKS:
   Morning:
   Afternoon:
   Evening:

Net Carbs: _____

Glasses of Water: _____

Let's Get Physical: _____
_____
_____
_____

How Am I Doing?: _____
_____
_____
_____

FRIDAY

Date: _____

Total Daily Net Carb Intake: _____

BREAKFAST:

Net Carbs: _____

LUNCH:

Net Carbs: _____

DINNER:

Net Carbs: _____

SNACKS:
  Morning:
  Afternoon:
  Evening:

Net Carbs: _____

Glasses of Water: _____

Let's Get Physical: _____

_____

_____

How Am I Doing?: _____

_____

_____

SATURDAY

Date: _____

Total Daily Net Carb Intake: _____

BREAKFAST:

Net Carbs: _____

LUNCH:

Net Carbs: _____

DINNER:

Net Carbs: _____

SNACKS:
   Morning:
   Afternoon:
   Evening:

Net Carbs: _____

Glasses of Water: _____

Let's Get Physical: _____
_____
_____
_____

How Am I Doing?: _____
_____
_____
_____

WEEK TWO

Clean out your cupboards! Now that you're settling into your new low-carb lifestyle, remove all temptations. Collect your high-carb foods—white flour, white bread, white rice, pasta, cookies, doughnuts, muffins, cakes, pies, croissants, potato chips, soda, etc.—and donate them to a local food bank or shelter.

Instead stock up on healthy low-carb snacks, such as protein bars, nuts, seeds, fresh olives, jars of marinated artichokes, roasted red peppers, avocados, salad greens, berries, soy chips, eggs, canned tuna, cheese, and unprocessed cold cuts (for example, fresh turkey breast and roast beef).

Daily Carb Quota: _____

SUNDAY

Date: _____

Total Daily Net Carb Intake: _____

BREAKFAST:

Net Carbs: _____

LUNCH:

Net Carbs: _____

DINNER:

Net Carbs: _____

SNACKS:
  Morning:
  Afternoon:
  Evening:

Net Carbs: _____

Glasses of Water: _____

Let's Get Physical: _____
_____
_____
_____

How Am I Doing?: _____
_____
_____
_____

MONDAY

Date: _____

Total Daily Net Carb Intake: _____

BREAKFAST:

Net Carbs: _____

LUNCH:

Net Carbs: _____

DINNER:

Net Carbs: _____

SNACKS:
   Morning:
   Afternoon:
   Evening:

Net Carbs: _____

Glasses of Water: _____

Let's Get Physical: _____
_____
_____
_____

How Am I Doing?: _____
_____
_____
_____

TUESDAY

Date: _____

Total Daily Net Carb Intake: _____

BREAKFAST:

Net Carbs: _____

LUNCH:

Net Carbs: _____

DINNER:

Net Carbs: _____

SNACKS:
　　Morning:
　　Afternoon:
　　Evening:

Net Carbs: _____

Glasses of Water: _____

Let's Get Physical: _____
_____
_____
_____

How Am I Doing?: _____
_____
_____
_____

WEDNESDAY

Date: _____

Total Daily Net Carb Intake: _____

BREAKFAST:

Net Carbs: _____

LUNCH:

Net Carbs: _____

DINNER:

Net Carbs: _____

SNACKS:
  Morning:
  Afternoon:
  Evening:

Net Carbs: _____

Glasses of Water: _____

Let's Get Physical: _____
_____
_____
_____

How Am I Doing?: _____
_____
_____
_____

THURSDAY

Date: _____

Total Daily Net Carb Intake: _____

BREAKFAST:

Net Carbs: _____

LUNCH:

Net Carbs: _____

DINNER:

Net Carbs: _____

SNACKS:
   Morning:
   Afternoon:
   Evening:

Net Carbs: _____

Glasses of Water: _____

Let's Get Physical: _____
_____
_____
_____

How Am I Doing?: _____
_____
_____
_____

FRIDAY

Date: _____

Total Daily Net Carb Intake: _____

BREAKFAST:

Net Carbs: _____

LUNCH:

Net Carbs: _____

DINNER:

Net Carbs: _____

SNACKS:
   Morning:
   Afternoon:
   Evening:
Net Carbs: _____

Glasses of Water: _____

Let's Get Physical: _____
_____
_____
_____

How Am I Doing?: _____
_____
_____
_____

SATURDAY

Date: _____

Total Daily Net Carb Intake: _____

BREAKFAST:

Net Carbs: _____

LUNCH:

Net Carbs: _____

DINNER:

Net Carbs: _____

SNACKS:
   Morning:
   Afternoon:
   Evening:

Net Carbs: _____

Glasses of Water: _____

Let's Get Physical: _____
_____
_____
_____

How Am I Doing?: _____
_____
_____
_____

WEEK THREE

Get moving! Exercise plays an important role in any diet plan, and even modest amounts—as little as 20 to 30 minutes three or four times a week—can help you control weight and improve your health overall. As your stamina improves, you can increase your exercise.

Of course, before you begin any new physical fitness program, it's important to see your physician. And as you begin to work out, listen to your body. If you have not exercised for some time, take it slow and take care not to overdo. If you feel any pain or unusual fatigue, take a break.

Daily Carb Quota: _____

SUNDAY

Date: _____

Total Daily Net Carb Intake: _____

BREAKFAST:

Net Carbs: _____

LUNCH:

Net Carbs: _____

DINNER:

Net Carbs: _____

SNACKS:
  Morning:
  Afternoon:
  Evening:

Net Carbs: _____

Glasses of Water: _____

Let's Get Physical: _____
_____
_____
_____

How Am I Doing?: _____
_____
_____
_____

MONDAY

Date: _____

Total Daily Net Carb Intake: _____

BREAKFAST:

Net Carbs: _____

LUNCH:

Net Carbs: _____

DINNER:

Net Carbs: _____

SNACKS:
  Morning:
  Afternoon:
  Evening:

Net Carbs: _____

Glasses of Water: _____

Let's Get Physical: _____
_____
_____
_____

How Am I Doing?: _____
_____
_____
_____

TUESDAY

Date: _____

Total Daily Net Carb Intake: _____

BREAKFAST:

Net Carbs: _____

LUNCH:

Net Carbs: _____

DINNER:

Net Carbs: _____

SNACKS:
　Morning:
　Afternoon:
　Evening:

Net Carbs: _____

Glasses of Water: _____

Let's Get Physical: _____
_____
_____
_____

How Am I Doing?: _____
_____
_____
_____

WEDNESDAY

Date: _____

Total Daily Net Carb Intake: _____

BREAKFAST:

Net Carbs: _____

LUNCH:

Net Carbs: _____

DINNER:

Net Carbs: _____

SNACKS:
  Morning:
  Afternoon:
  Evening:

Net Carbs: _____

Glasses of Water: _____

Let's Get Physical: _____
_____
_____
_____

How Am I Doing?: _____
_____
_____
_____

THURSDAY

Date: _____

Total Daily Net Carb Intake: _____

BREAKFAST:

Net Carbs: _____

LUNCH:

Net Carbs: _____

DINNER:

Net Carbs: _____

SNACKS:
 Morning:
 Afternoon:
 Evening:

Net Carbs: _____

Glasses of Water: _____

Let's Get Physical: _____
_____
_____
_____

How Am I Doing?: _____
_____
_____
_____

FRIDAY

Date: _____

Total Daily Net Carb Intake: _____

BREAKFAST:

Net Carbs: _____

LUNCH:

Net Carbs: _____

DINNER:

Net Carbs: _____

SNACKS:
   Morning:
   Afternoon:
   Evening:

Net Carbs: _____

Glasses of Water: _____

Let's Get Physical: _____
_____
_____
_____

How Am I Doing?: _____
_____
_____
_____

SATURDAY

Date: _____

Total Daily Net Carb Intake: _____

BREAKFAST:

Net Carbs: _____

LUNCH:

Net Carbs: _____

DINNER:

Net Carbs: _____

SNACKS:
   Morning:
   Afternoon:
   Evening:

Net Carbs: _____

Glasses of Water: _____

Let's Get Physical: _____
_____
_____
_____

How Am I Doing?: _____
_____
_____
_____

WEEK FOUR

Lose your fear of fat! Remember that it's the carbs you want to focus on now. Moreover, products labeled as low-fat usually don't include significantly less fat than their full-fat counterparts. You can now enjoy healthy fats such as olive oil and nuts without guilt. So reach for a handful of satisfying nuts when you crave a snack and enjoy full-fat dressings on your salad (with an ounce of cheese for good measure). Equally important, stay away from processed foods labelled "low-fat"—especially baked goods and low-fat ice cream. To make up for the missing flavor provided by fat, manufacturers typically pile on the sugar—and extra carbs—which is exactly what you *don't* want.

Daily Carb Quota: _____

SUNDAY

Date: _____

Total Daily Net Carb Intake: _____

BREAKFAST:

Net Carbs: _____

LUNCH:

Net Carbs: _____

DINNER:

Net Carbs: _____

SNACKS:
  Morning:
  Afternoon:
  Evening:

Net Carbs: _____

Glasses of Water: _____

Let's Get Physical: _____
_____
_____
_____

How Am I Doing?: _____
_____
_____
_____

MONDAY

Date: _____

Total Daily Net Carb Intake: _____

BREAKFAST:

Net Carbs: _____

LUNCH:

Net Carbs: _____

DINNER:

Net Carbs: _____

SNACKS:
  Morning:
  Afternoon:
  Evening:

Net Carbs: _____

Glasses of Water: _____

Let's Get Physical: _____
_____
_____
_____

How Am I Doing?: _____
_____
_____
_____

TUESDAY

Date: _____

Total Daily Net Carb Intake: _____

BREAKFAST:

Net Carbs: _____

LUNCH:

Net Carbs: _____

DINNER:

Net Carbs: _____

SNACKS:
   Morning:
   Afternoon:
   Evening:

Net Carbs: _____

Glasses of Water: _____

Let's Get Physical: _____
_____
_____
_____

How Am I Doing?: _____
_____
_____
_____

WEDNESDAY

Date: _____

Total Daily Net Carb Intake: _____

BREAKFAST:

Net Carbs: _____

LUNCH:

Net Carbs: _____

DINNER:

Net Carbs: _____

SNACKS:
  Morning:
  Afternoon:
  Evening:

Net Carbs: _____

Glasses of Water: _____

Let's Get Physical: _____
_____
_____

How Am I Doing?: _____
_____
_____
_____

THURSDAY

Date: _____

Total Daily Net Carb Intake: _____

BREAKFAST:

Net Carbs: _____

LUNCH:

Net Carbs: _____

DINNER:

Net Carbs: _____

SNACKS:
   Morning:
   Afternoon:
   Evening:

Net Carbs: _____

Glasses of Water: _____

Let's Get Physical: _____
_____
_____
_____

How Am I Doing?: _____
_____
_____
_____

FRIDAY

Date: _____

Total Daily Net Carb Intake: _____

BREAKFAST:

Net Carbs: _____

LUNCH:

Net Carbs: _____

DINNER:

Net Carbs: _____

SNACKS:
  Morning:
  Afternoon:
  Evening:

Net Carbs: _____

Glasses of Water: _____

Let's Get Physical: _____
_____
_____
_____

How Am I Doing?: _____
_____
_____
_____

SATURDAY

Date: _____

Total Daily Net Carb Intake: _____

BREAKFAST:

Net Carbs: _____

LUNCH:

Net Carbs: _____

DINNER:

Net Carbs: _____

SNACKS:
   Morning:
   Afternoon:
   Evening:

Net Carbs: _____

Glasses of Water: _____

Let's Get Physical: _____
_____
_____
_____

How Am I Doing?: _____
_____
_____
_____

WEEK FIVE

Congratulations! You have completed four weeks of your new low-carb lifestyle, and it's time to take a step back and look at the big picture. Are you losing weight yet? Do you have more energy? Do you feel better overall? If the answers are yes, great. If not, don't give up.

Are you watching out for hidden carbs? Salad dressings, sauces, and gravies often contain white flour or sugar—and these can be your undoing. Read labels, consult your carb counter, and choose low-carb alternatives.

And are you taking a daily vitamin and mineral supplement? Whatever diet plan you choose, it is essential that you get your daily requirement of vitamins and minerals.

Look back in your diary to review your food selections and the challenges you've faced in the last four weeks. Don't be hard on yourself if you haven't always made the best choices, but do come up with more positive coping strategies for the future. For example, arm yourself against the peril of late-afternoon snack attacks! Tuck a package of nuts or a low-carb protein bar into your pocketbook or briefcase. This way you won't be tempted to stop at the candy or chips machine.

Daily Carb Quota: _____

SUNDAY

Date: _____

Total Daily Net Carb Intake: _____

BREAKFAST:

Net Carbs: _____

LUNCH:

Net Carbs: _____

DINNER:

Net Carbs: _____

SNACKS:
   Morning:
   Afternoon:
   Evening:

Net Carbs: _____

Glasses of Water: _____

Let's Get Physical: _____
_____
_____
_____

How Am I Doing?: _____
_____
_____
_____

MONDAY

Date: _____

Total Daily Net Carb Intake: _____

BREAKFAST:

Net Carbs: _____

LUNCH:

Net Carbs: _____

DINNER:

Net Carbs: _____

SNACKS:
   Morning:
   Afternoon:
   Evening:

Net Carbs: _____

Glasses of Water: _____

Let's Get Physical: _____
_____
_____
_____

How Am I Doing?: _____
_____
_____
_____

TUESDAY

Date: _____

Total Daily Net Carb Intake: _____

BREAKFAST:

Net Carbs: _____

LUNCH:

Net Carbs: _____

DINNER:

Net Carbs: _____

SNACKS:
   Morning:
   Afternoon:
   Evening:

Net Carbs: _____

Glasses of Water: _____

Let's Get Physical: _____
_____
_____
_____

How Am I Doing?: _____
_____
_____
_____

WEDNESDAY

Date: _____

Total Daily Net Carb Intake: _____

BREAKFAST:

Net Carbs: _____

LUNCH:

Net Carbs: _____

DINNER:

Net Carbs: _____

SNACKS:
    Morning:
    Afternoon:
    Evening:

Net Carbs: _____

Glasses of Water: _____

Let's Get Physical: _____
_____
_____
_____

How Am I Doing?: _____
_____
_____
_____

THURSDAY

Date: _____

Total Daily Net Carb Intake: _____

BREAKFAST:

Net Carbs: _____

LUNCH:

Net Carbs: _____

DINNER:

Net Carbs: _____

SNACKS:
   Morning:
   Afternoon:
   Evening:

Net Carbs: _____

Glasses of Water: _____

Let's Get Physical: _____
_____
_____
_____

How Am I Doing?: _____
_____
_____
_____

FRIDAY

Date: _____

Total Daily Net Carb Intake: _____

BREAKFAST:

Net Carbs: _____

LUNCH:

Net Carbs: _____

DINNER:

Net Carbs: _____

SNACKS:
   Morning:
   Afternoon:
   Evening:

Net Carbs: _____

Glasses of Water: _____

Let's Get Physical: _____
_____
_____
_____

How Am I Doing?: _____
_____
_____
_____

SATURDAY

Date: _____

Total Daily Net Carb Intake: _____

BREAKFAST:

Net Carbs: _____

LUNCH:

Net Carbs: _____

DINNER:

Net Carbs: _____

SNACKS:
    Morning:
    Afternoon:
    Evening:

Net Carbs: _____

Glasses of Water: _____

Let's Get Physical: _____
_____
_____
_____

How Am I Doing?: _____
_____
_____
_____

WEEK SIX

Drink up! Water is the healthiest beverage around. It helps you to flush the toxins from your body and avoid dehydration and constipation. Your goal is to drink eight 8-ounce glasses every day. Remember to keep track of daily water consumption in your diary.

Daily Carb Quota: _____

SUNDAY

Date: _____

Total Daily Net Carb Intake: _____

BREAKFAST:

Net Carbs: _____

LUNCH:

Net Carbs: _____

DINNER:

Net Carbs: _____

SNACKS:
  Morning:
  Afternoon:
  Evening:

Net Carbs: _____

Glasses of Water: _____

Let's Get Physical: _____
_____
_____
_____

How Am I Doing?: _____
_____
_____
_____

MONDAY

Date: _____

Total Daily Net Carb Intake: _____

BREAKFAST:

Net Carbs: _____

LUNCH:

Net Carbs: _____

DINNER:

Net Carbs: _____

SNACKS:
  Morning:
  Afternoon:
  Evening:

Net Carbs: _____

Glasses of Water: _____

Let's Get Physical: _____
_____
_____
_____

How Am I Doing?: _____
_____
_____
_____

TUESDAY

Date: _____

Total Daily Net Carb Intake: _____

BREAKFAST:

Net Carbs: _____

LUNCH:

Net Carbs: _____

DINNER:

Net Carbs: _____

SNACKS:
  Morning:
  Afternoon:
  Evening:

Net Carbs: _____

Glasses of Water: _____

Let's Get Physical: _____
_____
_____
_____

How Am I Doing?: _____
_____
_____
_____

WEDNESDAY

Date: _____

Total Daily Net Carb Intake: _____

BREAKFAST:

Net Carbs: _____

LUNCH:

Net Carbs: _____

DINNER:

Net Carbs: _____

SNACKS:
   Morning:
   Afternoon:
   Evening:

Net Carbs: _____

Glasses of Water: _____

Let's Get Physical: _____
_____
_____
_____

How Am I Doing?: _____
_____
_____
_____

THURSDAY

Date: _____

Total Daily Net Carb Intake: _____

BREAKFAST:

Net Carbs: _____

LUNCH:

Net Carbs: _____

DINNER:

Net Carbs: _____

SNACKS:
 Morning:
 Afternoon:
 Evening:

Net Carbs: _____

Glasses of Water: _____

Let's Get Physical: _____
_____
_____
_____

How Am I Doing?: _____
_____
_____
_____

FRIDAY

Date: _____

Total Daily Net Carb Intake: _____

BREAKFAST:

Net Carbs: _____

LUNCH:

Net Carbs: _____

DINNER:

Net Carbs: _____

SNACKS:
   Morning:
   Afternoon:
   Evening:

Net Carbs: _____

Glasses of Water: _____

Let's Get Physical: _____
_____
_____
_____

How Am I Doing?: _____
_____
_____
_____

SATURDAY

Date: _____

Total Daily Net Carb Intake: _____

BREAKFAST:

Net Carbs: _____

LUNCH:

Net Carbs: _____

DINNER:

Net Carbs: _____

SNACKS:
   Morning:
   Afternoon:
   Evening:

Net Carbs: _____

Glasses of Water: _____

Let's Get Physical: _____
_____
_____
_____

How Am I Doing?: _____
_____
_____
_____

WEEK SEVEN

Go fishing! Or just visit your local market to choose fish or shellfish for dinner tonight. Not only are they low in carbs, many fish—such as salmon, mackerel, sardines, trout, and tuna—are packed with heart-healthy omega-3 fatty acids.

Daily Carb Quota: _____

SUNDAY

Date: _____

Total Daily Net Carb Intake: _____

BREAKFAST:

Net Carbs: _____

LUNCH:

Net Carbs: _____

DINNER:

Net Carbs: _____

SNACKS:
   Morning:
   Afternoon:
   Evening:

Net Carbs: _____

Glasses of Water: _____

Let's Get Physical: _____
_____
_____
_____

How Am I Doing?: _____
_____
_____
_____

MONDAY

Date: _____

Total Daily Net Carb Intake: _____

BREAKFAST:

Net Carbs: _____

LUNCH:

Net Carbs: _____

DINNER:

Net Carbs: _____

SNACKS:
   Morning:
   Afternoon:
   Evening:

Net Carbs: _____

Glasses of Water: _____

Let's Get Physical: _____
_____
_____
_____

How Am I Doing?: _____
_____
_____
_____

TUESDAY

Date: _____

Total Daily Net Carb Intake: _____

BREAKFAST:

Net Carbs: _____

LUNCH:

Net Carbs: _____

DINNER:

Net Carbs: _____

SNACKS:
  Morning:
  Afternoon:
  Evening:

Net Carbs: _____

Glasses of Water: _____

Let's Get Physical: _____
_____
_____
_____

How Am I Doing?: _____
_____
_____
_____

WEDNESDAY

Date: _____

Total Daily Net Carb Intake: _____

BREAKFAST:

Net Carbs: _____

LUNCH:

Net Carbs: _____

DINNER:

Net Carbs: _____

SNACKS:
   Morning:
   Afternoon:
   Evening:

Net Carbs: _____

Glasses of Water: _____

Let's Get Physical: _____

_____
_____
_____

How Am I Doing?: _____

_____
_____
_____

THURSDAY

Date: _____

Total Daily Net Carb Intake: _____

BREAKFAST:

Net Carbs: _____

LUNCH:

Net Carbs: _____

DINNER:

Net Carbs: _____

SNACKS:
  Morning:
  Afternoon:
  Evening:

Net Carbs: _____

Glasses of Water: _____

Let's Get Physical: _____
_____
_____
_____

How Am I Doing?: _____
_____
_____
_____

FRIDAY

Date: _____

Total Daily Net Carb Intake: _____

BREAKFAST:

Net Carbs: _____

LUNCH:

Net Carbs: _____

DINNER:

Net Carbs: _____

SNACKS:
   Morning:
   Afternoon:
   Evening:

Net Carbs: _____

Glasses of Water: _____

Let's Get Physical: _____

_____

_____

_____

How Am I Doing?: _____

_____

_____

_____

SATURDAY

Date: _____

Total Daily Net Carb Intake: _____

BREAKFAST:

Net Carbs: _____

LUNCH:

Net Carbs: _____

DINNER:

Net Carbs: _____

SNACKS:
  Morning:
  Afternoon:
  Evening:

Net Carbs: _____

Glasses of Water: _____

Let's Get Physical: _____
_____
_____
_____

How Am I Doing?: _____
_____
_____
_____

WEEK EIGHT

When you do your weekly shopping at the local grocery store, stick to the outer aisles. There you'll find whole foods such as fresh veggies, fruit, seafood, meats, cheeses, and other dairy items. Don't allow yourself to be seduced into the inner aisles, which are stocked with processed foods high in carbs, sodium, and trans fats. Whenever you go shopping, read labels, and look up carb counts in your carb counter.

Daily Carb Quota: _____

SUNDAY

Date: _____

Total Daily Net Carb Intake: _____

BREAKFAST:

Net Carbs: _____

LUNCH:

Net Carbs: _____

DINNER:

Net Carbs: _____

SNACKS:
  Morning:
  Afternoon:
  Evening:

Net Carbs: _____

Glasses of Water: _____

Let's Get Physical: _____
_____
_____
_____

How Am I Doing?: _____
_____
_____
_____

MONDAY

Date: _____

Total Daily Net Carb Intake: _____

BREAKFAST:

Net Carbs: _____

LUNCH:

Net Carbs: _____

DINNER:

Net Carbs: _____

SNACKS:
  Morning:
  Afternoon:
  Evening:

Net Carbs: _____

Glasses of Water: _____

Let's Get Physical: _____
_____
_____
_____

How Am I Doing?: _____
_____
_____
_____

TUESDAY

Date: _____

Total Daily Net Carb Intake: _____

BREAKFAST:

Net Carbs: _____

LUNCH:

Net Carbs: _____

DINNER:

Net Carbs: _____

SNACKS:
   Morning:
   Afternoon:
   Evening:

Net Carbs: _____

Glasses of Water: _____

Let's Get Physical: _____
_____
_____
_____

How Am I Doing?: _____
_____
_____
_____

WEDNESDAY

Date: _____

Total Daily Net Carb Intake: _____

BREAKFAST:

Net Carbs: _____

LUNCH:

Net Carbs: _____

DINNER:

Net Carbs: _____

SNACKS:
    Morning:
    Afternoon:
    Evening:

Net Carbs: _____

Glasses of Water: _____

Let's Get Physical: _____
_____
_____
_____

How Am I Doing?: _____
_____
_____
_____

THURSDAY

Date: _____

Total Daily Net Carb Intake: _____

BREAKFAST:

Net Carbs: _____

LUNCH:

Net Carbs: _____

DINNER:

Net Carbs: _____

SNACKS:
 Morning:
 Afternoon:
 Evening:

Net Carbs: _____

Glasses of Water: _____

Let's Get Physical: _____
_____
_____
_____

How Am I Doing?: _____
_____
_____
_____

FRIDAY

Date: _____

Total Daily Net Carb Intake: _____

BREAKFAST:

Net Carbs: _____

LUNCH:

Net Carbs: _____

DINNER:

Net Carbs: _____

SNACKS:
   Morning:
   Afternoon:
   Evening:

Net Carbs: _____

Glasses of Water: _____

Let's Get Physical: _____
_____
_____
_____

How Am I Doing?: _____
_____
_____
_____

SATURDAY

Date: _____

Total Daily Net Carb Intake: _____

BREAKFAST:

Net Carbs: _____

LUNCH:

Net Carbs: _____

DINNER:

Net Carbs: _____

SNACKS:
  Morning:
  Afternoon:
  Evening:

Net Carbs: _____

Glasses of Water: _____

Let's Get Physical: _____
_____
_____
_____

How Am I Doing?: _____
_____
_____
_____

WEEK NINE

Congratulations! You've now completed eight weeks of your new low-carb lifestyle. So how are you doing? Are you keeping track? Don't limit your diary entries to carb counts alone. Each night before you go to sleep, also jot down your accomplishments for the day—that brisk walk you took in the morning with a friend, how you used the stairs instead of the elevator, the carbs you so successfully steered clear of at the company party.

At the end of each week, review your accomplishments and give yourself a pat on the back. Think about indulging in a well-deserved reward (as long as it's not food!). Maybe a new outfit in a smaller size, a massage, a night out dancing, or taking in a movie with friends.

Daily Carb Quota: _____

SUNDAY

Date: _____

Total Daily Net Carb Intake: _____

BREAKFAST:

Net Carbs: _____

LUNCH:

Net Carbs: _____

DINNER:

Net Carbs: _____

SNACKS:
   Morning:
   Afternoon:
   Evening:

Net Carbs: _____

Glasses of Water: _____

Let's Get Physical: _____
_____
_____
_____

How Am I Doing?: _____
_____
_____
_____

MONDAY

Date: _____

Total Daily Net Carb Intake: _____

BREAKFAST:

Net Carbs: _____

LUNCH:

Net Carbs: _____

DINNER:

Net Carbs: _____

SNACKS:
   Morning:
   Afternoon:
   Evening:

Net Carbs: _____

Glasses of Water: _____

Let's Get Physical: _____
_____
_____
_____

How Am I Doing?: _____
_____
_____
_____

TUESDAY

Date: _____

Total Daily Net Carb Intake: _____

BREAKFAST:

Net Carbs: _____

LUNCH:

Net Carbs: _____

DINNER:

Net Carbs: _____

SNACKS:
   Morning:
   Afternoon:
   Evening:

Net Carbs: _____

Glasses of Water: _____

Let's Get Physical: _____
_____
_____
_____

How Am I Doing?: _____
_____
_____
_____

WEDNESDAY

Date: _____

Total Daily Net Carb Intake: _____

BREAKFAST:

Net Carbs: _____

LUNCH:

Net Carbs: _____

DINNER:

Net Carbs: _____

SNACKS:
   Morning:
   Afternoon:
   Evening:

Net Carbs: _____

Glasses of Water: _____

Let's Get Physical: _____
_____
_____
_____

How Am I Doing?: _____
_____
_____
_____

THURSDAY

Date: _____

Total Daily Net Carb Intake: _____

BREAKFAST:

Net Carbs: _____

LUNCH:

Net Carbs: _____

DINNER:

Net Carbs: _____

SNACKS:
 Morning:
 Afternoon:
 Evening:

Net Carbs: _____

Glasses of Water: _____

Let's Get Physical: _____
_____
_____
_____

How Am I Doing?: _____
_____
_____
_____

FRIDAY

Date: _____

Total Daily Net Carb Intake: _____

BREAKFAST:

Net Carbs: _____

LUNCH:

Net Carbs: _____

DINNER:

Net Carbs: _____

SNACKS:
   Morning:
   Afternoon:
   Evening:

Net Carbs: _____

Glasses of Water: _____

Let's Get Physical: _____
_____
_____
_____

How Am I Doing?: _____
_____
_____
_____

SATURDAY

Date: _____

Total Daily Net Carb Intake: _____

BREAKFAST:

Net Carbs: _____

LUNCH:

Net Carbs: _____

DINNER:

Net Carbs: _____

SNACKS:
    Morning:
    Afternoon:
    Evening:

Net Carbs: _____

Glasses of Water: _____

Let's Get Physical: _____
_____
_____
_____

How Am I Doing?: _____
_____
_____
_____

WEEK TEN

When you choose a salad as your main course, do both your palate and your metabolism a favor by topping it with grilled fish, steak, or chicken. Not only will your meal feel more satisfying, the added protein and fat will slow the impact of carbs on blood sugar.

Daily Carb Quota: _____

SUNDAY

Date: _____

Total Daily Net Carb Intake: _____

BREAKFAST:

Net Carbs: _____

LUNCH:

Net Carbs: _____

DINNER:

Net Carbs: _____

SNACKS:
　　Morning:
　　Afternoon:
　　Evening:

Net Carbs: _____

Glasses of Water: _____

Let's Get Physical: _____
_____
_____
_____

How Am I Doing?: _____
_____
_____
_____

MONDAY

Date: _____

Total Daily Net Carb Intake: _____

BREAKFAST:

Net Carbs: _____

LUNCH:

Net Carbs: _____

DINNER:

Net Carbs: _____

SNACKS:
  Morning:
  Afternoon:
  Evening:

Net Carbs: _____

Glasses of Water: _____

Let's Get Physical: _____
_____
_____
_____

How Am I Doing?: _____
_____
_____
_____

TUESDAY

Date: _____

Total Daily Net Carb Intake: _____

BREAKFAST:

Net Carbs: _____

LUNCH:

Net Carbs: _____

DINNER:

Net Carbs: _____

SNACKS:
  Morning:
  Afternoon:
  Evening:

Net Carbs: _____

Glasses of Water: _____

Let's Get Physical: _____
_____
_____
_____

How Am I Doing?: _____
_____
_____
_____

WEDNESDAY

Date: _____

Total Daily Net Carb Intake: _____

BREAKFAST:

Net Carbs: _____

LUNCH:

Net Carbs: _____

DINNER:

Net Carbs: _____

SNACKS:
  Morning:
  Afternoon:
  Evening:

Net Carbs: _____

Glasses of Water: _____

Let's Get Physical: _____

_____

_____

How Am I Doing?: _____

_____

_____

THURSDAY

Date: _____

Total Daily Net Carb Intake: _____

BREAKFAST:

Net Carbs: _____

LUNCH:

Net Carbs: _____

DINNER:

Net Carbs: _____

SNACKS:
    Morning:
    Afternoon:
    Evening:

Net Carbs: _____

Glasses of Water: _____

Let's Get Physical: _____
_____
_____
_____

How Am I Doing?: _____
_____
_____
_____

FRIDAY

Date: _____

Total Daily Net Carb Intake: _____

BREAKFAST:

Net Carbs: _____

LUNCH:

Net Carbs: _____

DINNER:

Net Carbs: _____

SNACKS:
   Morning:
   Afternoon:
   Evening:
Net Carbs: _____

Glasses of Water: _____

Let's Get Physical: _____
_____
_____
_____

How Am I Doing?: _____
_____
_____
_____

SATURDAY

Date: _____

Total Daily Net Carb Intake: _____

BREAKFAST:

Net Carbs: _____

LUNCH:

Net Carbs: _____

DINNER:

Net Carbs: _____

SNACKS:
Morning:
Afternoon:
Evening:

Net Carbs: _____

Glasses of Water: _____

Let's Get Physical: _____
_____
_____
_____

How Am I Doing?: _____
_____
_____
_____

WEEK ELEVEN

Don't skip meals! When you get very hungry, you're liable to reach for any old food to satisfy your craving. Eating small, regular meals—including snacks—gives you more control over your diet and keeps your blood sugar on an even keel.

Daily Carb Quota: _____

SUNDAY

Date: _____

Total Daily Net Carb Intake: _____

BREAKFAST:

Net Carbs: _____

LUNCH:

Net Carbs: _____

DINNER:

Net Carbs: _____

SNACKS:
  Morning:
  Afternoon:
  Evening:

Net Carbs: _____

Glasses of Water: _____

Let's Get Physical: _____
_____
_____
_____

How Am I Doing?: _____
_____
_____
_____

MONDAY

Date: _____

Total Daily Net Carb Intake: _____

BREAKFAST:

Net Carbs: _____

LUNCH:

Net Carbs: _____

DINNER:

Net Carbs: _____

SNACKS:
   Morning:
   Afternoon:
   Evening:

Net Carbs: _____

Glasses of Water: _____

Let's Get Physical: _____
_____
_____
_____

How Am I Doing?: _____
_____
_____
_____

TUESDAY

Date: _____

Total Daily Net Carb Intake: _____

BREAKFAST:

Net Carbs: _____

LUNCH:

Net Carbs: _____

DINNER:

Net Carbs: _____

SNACKS:
   Morning:
   Afternoon:
   Evening:

Net Carbs: _____

Glasses of Water: _____

Let's Get Physical: _____
_____
_____
_____

How Am I Doing?: _____
_____
_____
_____

WEDNESDAY

Date: _____

Total Daily Net Carb Intake: _____

BREAKFAST:

Net Carbs: _____

LUNCH:

Net Carbs: _____

DINNER:

Net Carbs: _____

SNACKS:
   Morning:
   Afternoon:
   Evening:

Net Carbs: _____

Glasses of Water: _____

Let's Get Physical: _____
_____
_____
_____

How Am I Doing?: _____
_____
_____
_____

THURSDAY

Date: _____

Total Daily Net Carb Intake: _____

BREAKFAST:

Net Carbs: _____

LUNCH:

Net Carbs: _____

DINNER:

Net Carbs: _____

SNACKS:
   Morning:
   Afternoon:
   Evening:

Net Carbs: _____

Glasses of Water: _____

Let's Get Physical: _____
_____
_____
_____

How Am I Doing?: _____
_____
_____
_____

FRIDAY

Date: _____

Total Daily Net Carb Intake: _____

BREAKFAST:

Net Carbs: _____

LUNCH:

Net Carbs: _____

DINNER:

Net Carbs: _____

SNACKS:
  Morning:
  Afternoon:
  Evening:

Net Carbs: _____

Glasses of Water: _____

Let's Get Physical: _____
_____
_____
_____

How Am I Doing?: _____
_____
_____
_____

SATURDAY

Date: _____

Total Daily Net Carb Intake: _____

BREAKFAST:

Net Carbs: _____

LUNCH:

Net Carbs: _____

DINNER:

Net Carbs: _____

SNACKS:
  Morning:
  Afternoon:
  Evening:

Net Carbs: _____

Glasses of Water: _____

Let's Get Physical: _____
_____
_____
_____

How Am I Doing?: _____
_____
_____
_____

WEEK TWELVE

Meat and poultry are virtually carb free and are an important part of your new low-carb lifestyle. Just watch out for sauces and marinades, which may contain white flour, sugar, or cornstarch. Also beware of luncheon meats—such as bologna, liverwurst, and olive loaf—that are processed with fillers and contain carbs.

Daily Carb Quota: _____

SUNDAY

Date: _____

Total Daily Net Carb Intake: _____

BREAKFAST:

Net Carbs: _____

LUNCH:

Net Carbs: _____

DINNER:

Net Carbs: _____

SNACKS:
  Morning:
  Afternoon:
  Evening:

Net Carbs: _____

Glasses of Water: _____

Let's Get Physical: _____
_____
_____
_____

How Am I Doing?: _____
_____
_____
_____

MONDAY

Date: _____

Total Daily Net Carb Intake: _____

BREAKFAST:

Net Carbs: _____

LUNCH:

Net Carbs: _____

DINNER:

Net Carbs: _____

SNACKS:
   Morning:
   Afternoon:
   Evening:

Net Carbs: _____

Glasses of Water: _____

Let's Get Physical: _____
_____
_____
_____

How Am I Doing?: _____
_____
_____
_____

TUESDAY

Date: _____

Total Daily Net Carb Intake: _____

BREAKFAST:

Net Carbs: _____

LUNCH:

Net Carbs: _____

DINNER:

Net Carbs: _____

SNACKS:
  Morning:
  Afternoon:
  Evening:

Net Carbs: _____

Glasses of Water: _____

Let's Get Physical: _____
_____
_____
_____

How Am I Doing?: _____
_____
_____
_____

WEDNESDAY

Date: _____

Total Daily Net Carb Intake: _____

BREAKFAST:

Net Carbs: _____

LUNCH:

Net Carbs: _____

DINNER:

Net Carbs: _____

SNACKS:
  Morning:
  Afternoon:
  Evening:

Net Carbs: _____

Glasses of Water: _____

Let's Get Physical: _____
_____
_____
_____

How Am I Doing?: _____
_____
_____
_____

THURSDAY

Date: _____

Total Daily Net Carb Intake: _____

BREAKFAST:

Net Carbs: _____

LUNCH:

Net Carbs: _____

DINNER:

Net Carbs: _____

SNACKS:
   Morning:
   Afternoon:
   Evening:

Net Carbs: _____

Glasses of Water: _____

Let's Get Physical: _____
_____
_____
_____

How Am I Doing?: _____
_____
_____
_____

FRIDAY

Date: _____

Total Daily Net Carb Intake: _____

BREAKFAST:

Net Carbs: _____

LUNCH:

Net Carbs: _____

DINNER:

Net Carbs: _____

SNACKS:
   Morning:
   Afternoon:
   Evening:

Net Carbs: _____

Glasses of Water: _____

Let's Get Physical: _____
_____
_____
_____

How Am I Doing?: _____
_____
_____
_____

SATURDAY

Date: _____

Total Daily Net Carb Intake: _____

BREAKFAST:

Net Carbs: _____

LUNCH:

Net Carbs: _____

DINNER:

Net Carbs: _____

SNACKS:
　　Morning:
　　Afternoon:
　　Evening:

Net Carbs: _____

Glasses of Water: _____

Let's Get Physical: _____
_____
_____
_____

How Am I Doing?: _____
_____
_____
_____

WEEK THIRTEEN

Congratulations! You've reached the halfway point on your journey to a fitter and healthier new you. At this point, take a moment to enjoy a look back on all you've achieved. Since you've recorded daily entries in *Your Carb Diary*, this is easy to do! If you've consistently followed your new low-carb lifestyle and engaged in regular exercise, chances are you've not only shed pounds and inches, you also look and feel better overall!

To get a sense of your progress, record your starting vital stats, your current stats, and your target stats below.

Starting Weight: _____

Current Weight: _____

Target Weight: _____

Starting Clothing Size: _____

Current Clothing Size: _____

Target Clothing Size: _____

Starting Waist Measurement: _____

Current Waist Measurement: _____

Target Waist Measurement: _____

Daily Carb Quota: _____

SUNDAY

Date: _____

Total Daily Net Carb Intake: _____

BREAKFAST:

Net Carbs: _____

LUNCH:

Net Carbs: _____

DINNER:

Net Carbs: _____

SNACKS:
  Morning:
  Afternoon:
  Evening:

Net Carbs: _____

Glasses of Water: _____

Let's Get Physical: _____
_____
_____
_____

How Am I Doing?: _____
_____
_____
_____

MONDAY

Date: _____

Total Daily Net Carb Intake: _____

BREAKFAST:

Net Carbs: _____

LUNCH:

Net Carbs: _____

DiNNER:

Net Carbs: _____

SNACKS:
    Morning:
    Afternoon:
    Evening:

Net Carbs: _____

Glasses of Water: _____

Let's Get Physical: _____
_____
_____
_____

How Am I Doing?: _____
_____
_____
_____

TUESDAY

Date: _____

Total Daily Net Carb Intake: _____

BREAKFAST:

Net Carbs: _____

LUNCH:

Net Carbs: _____

DINNER:

Net Carbs: _____

SNACKS:
   Morning:
   Afternoon:
   Evening:

Net Carbs: _____

Glasses of Water: _____

Let's Get Physical: _____
_____
_____
_____

How Am I Doing?: _____
_____
_____
_____

WEDNESDAY

Date: _____

Total Daily Net Carb Intake: _____

BREAKFAST:

Net Carbs: _____

LUNCH:

Net Carbs: _____

DINNER:

Net Carbs: _____

SNACKS:
  Morning:
  Afternoon:
  Evening:

Net Carbs: _____

Glasses of Water: _____

Let's Get Physical: _____
_____
_____
_____

How Am I Doing?: _____
_____
_____
_____

THURSDAY

Date: _____

Total Daily Net Carb Intake: _____

BREAKFAST:

Net Carbs: _____

LUNCH:

Net Carbs: _____

DINNER:

Net Carbs: _____

SNACKS:
  Morning:
  Afternoon:
  Evening:

Net Carbs: _____

Glasses of Water: _____

Let's Get Physical: _____
_____
_____
_____

How Am I Doing?: _____
_____
_____
_____

FRIDAY

Date: _____

Total Daily Net Carb Intake: _____

BREAKFAST:

Net Carbs: _____

LUNCH:

Net Carbs: _____

DINNER:

Net Carbs: _____

SNACKS:
  Morning:
  Afternoon:
  Evening:

Net Carbs: _____

Glasses of Water: _____

Let's Get Physical: _____
_____
_____
_____

How Am I Doing?: _____
_____
_____
_____

SATURDAY

Date: _____

Total Daily Net Carb Intake: _____

BREAKFAST:

Net Carbs: _____

LUNCH:

Net Carbs: _____

DINNER:

Net Carbs: _____

SNACKS:
   Morning:
   Afternoon:
   Evening:

Net Carbs: _____

Glasses of Water: _____

Let's Get Physical: _____
_____
_____
_____

How Am I Doing?: _____
_____
_____
_____

WEEK FOURTEEN

Are you getting bored with your diet? Do you miss bread and pasta? Visit the health food store to explore new controlled carb options. Going low-carb no longer means limiting yourself to an endless parade of grilled fish or chicken and salad. For a change, have a sandwich on low-carb bread. Other low-carb options include soy-based pasta, pancake mix, tortillas, soups, and sugar-free nut butters.

Daily Carb Quota: _____

SUNDAY

Date: _____

Total Daily Net Carb Intake: _____

BREAKFAST:

Net Carbs: _____

LUNCH:

Net Carbs: _____

DINNER:

Net Carbs: _____

SNACKS:
   Morning:
   Afternoon:
   Evening:

Net Carbs: _____

Glasses of Water: _____

Let's Get Physical: _____
_____
_____
_____

How Am I Doing?: _____
_____
_____
_____

MONDAY

Date: _____

Total Daily Net Carb Intake: _____

BREAKFAST:

Net Carbs: _____

LUNCH:

Net Carbs: _____

DINNER:

Net Carbs: _____

SNACKS:
    Morning:
    Afternoon:
    Evening:

Net Carbs: _____

Glasses of Water: _____

Let's Get Physical: _____
_____
_____
_____

How Am I Doing?: _____
_____
_____
_____

TUESDAY

Date: _____

Total Daily Net Carb Intake: _____

BREAKFAST:

Net Carbs: _____

LUNCH:

Net Carbs: _____

DINNER:

Net Carbs: _____

SNACKS:
    Morning:
    Afternoon:
    Evening:

Net Carbs: _____

Glasses of Water: _____

Let's Get Physical: _____
_____
_____
_____

How Am I Doing?: _____
_____
_____
_____

WEDNESDAY

Date: _____

Total Daily Net Carb Intake: _____

BREAKFAST:

Net Carbs: _____

LUNCH:

Net Carbs: _____

DINNER:

Net Carbs: _____

SNACKS:
  Morning:
  Afternoon:
  Evening:

Net Carbs: _____

Glasses of Water: _____

Let's Get Physical: _____
_____
_____
_____

How Am I Doing?: _____
_____
_____
_____

THURSDAY

Date: _____

Total Daily Net Carb Intake: _____

BREAKFAST:

Net Carbs: _____

LUNCH:

Net Carbs: _____

DINNER:

Net Carbs: _____

SNACKS:
  Morning:
  Afternoon:
  Evening:

Net Carbs: _____

Glasses of Water: _____

Let's Get Physical: _____
_____
_____
_____

How Am I Doing?: _____
_____
_____
_____

FRIDAY

Date: _____

Total Daily Net Carb Intake: _____

BREAKFAST:

Net Carbs: _____

LUNCH:

Net Carbs: _____

DINNER:

Net Carbs: _____

SNACKS:
   Morning:
   Afternoon:
   Evening:

Net Carbs: _____

Glasses of Water: _____

Let's Get Physical: _____

_____

_____

How Am I Doing?: _____

_____

_____

SATURDAY

Date: _____

Total Daily Net Carb Intake: _____

BREAKFAST:

Net Carbs: _____

LUNCH:

Net Carbs: _____

DINNER:

Net Carbs: _____

SNACKS:
  Morning:
  Afternoon:
  Evening:

Net Carbs: _____

Glasses of Water: _____

Let's Get Physical: _____
_____
_____
_____

How Am I Doing?: _____
_____
_____
_____

WEEK FIFTEEN

When dining out, you're the boss. After all, who's paying the bill? Don't be shy about asking how foods are prepared and giving instructions about how you'd like them. Helpful tips include asking for the dressing or sauce on the side, and replacing high-carb starches such as rice and potatoes with an extra serving of vegetables. Also keep in mind that your mother was wrong when she told you to clean your plate at each meal—eat until you're comfortably full and no more. Take any leftovers home in a doggie bag.

Daily Carb Quota: _____

SUNDAY

Date: _____

Total Daily Net Carb Intake: _____

BREAKFAST:

Net Carbs: _____

LUNCH:

Net Carbs: _____

DINNER:

Net Carbs: _____

SNACKS:
Morning:
Afternoon:
Evening:

Net Carbs: _____

Glasses of Water: _____

Let's Get Physical: _____
_____
_____
_____

How Am I Doing?: _____
_____
_____
_____

MONDAY

Date: _____

Total Daily Net Carb Intake: _____

BREAKFAST:

Net Carbs: _____

LUNCH:

Net Carbs: _____

DINNER:

Net Carbs: _____

SNACKS:
   Morning:
   Afternoon:
   Evening:

Net Carbs: _____

Glasses of Water: _____

Let's Get Physical: _____

_____

_____

_____

How Am I Doing?: _____

_____

_____

_____

TUESDAY

Date: _____

Total Daily Net Carb Intake: _____

BREAKFAST:

Net Carbs: _____

LUNCH:

Net Carbs: _____

DINNER:

Net Carbs: _____

SNACKS:
   Morning:
   Afternoon:
   Evening:

Net Carbs: _____

Glasses of Water: _____

Let's Get Physical: _____
_____
_____
_____

How Am I Doing?: _____
_____
_____
_____

WEDNESDAY

Date: _____

Total Daily Net Carb Intake: _____

BREAKFAST:

Net Carbs: _____

LUNCH:

Net Carbs: _____

DINNER:

Net Carbs: _____

SNACKS:
    Morning:
    Afternoon:
    Evening:

Net Carbs: _____

Glasses of Water: _____

Let's Get Physical: _____
_____
_____
_____

How Am I Doing?: _____
_____
_____
_____

THURSDAY

Date: _____

Total Daily Net Carb Intake: _____

BREAKFAST:

Net Carbs: _____

LUNCH:

Net Carbs: _____

DINNER:

Net Carbs: _____

SNACKS:
  Morning:
  Afternoon:
  Evening:

Net Carbs: _____

Glasses of Water: _____

Let's Get Physical: _____
_____
_____
_____

How Am I Doing?: _____
_____
_____
_____

FRIDAY

Date: _____

Total Daily Net Carb Intake: _____

BREAKFAST:

Net Carbs: _____

LUNCH:

Net Carbs: _____

DINNER:

Net Carbs: _____

SNACKS:
   Morning:
   Afternoon:
   Evening:

Net Carbs: _____

Glasses of Water: _____

Let's Get Physical: _____
_____
_____
_____

How Am I Doing?: _____
_____
_____
_____

SATURDAY

Date: _____

Total Daily Net Carb Intake: _____

BREAKFAST:

Net Carbs: _____

LUNCH:

Net Carbs: _____

DINNER:

Net Carbs: _____

SNACKS:
  Morning:
  Afternoon:
  Evening:

Net Carbs: _____

Glasses of Water: _____

Let's Get Physical: _____
_____
_____
_____

How Am I Doing?: _____
_____
_____
_____

WEEK SIXTEEN

Tasty, satisfying, and low in carbs, cheese is a great choice for a snack. But don't get greedy—stick to the small portion sizes noted in your carb counter. You can stretch small amounts by shredding or grating them. Avoid processed cheese foods or spreads, which are higher in carbs.

Daily Carb Quota: _____

SUNDAY

Date: _____

Total Daily Net Carb Intake: _____

BREAKFAST:

Net Carbs: _____

LUNCH:

Net Carbs: _____

DINNER:

Net Carbs: _____

SNACKS:
  Morning:
  Afternoon:
  Evening:

Net Carbs: _____

Glasses of Water: _____

Let's Get Physical: _____
_____
_____
_____

How Am I Doing?: _____
_____
_____
_____

MONDAY

Date: _____

Total Daily Net Carb Intake: _____

BREAKFAST:

Net Carbs: _____

LUNCH:

Net Carbs: _____

DINNER:

Net Carbs: _____

SNACKS:
   Morning:
   Afternoon:
   Evening:

Net Carbs: _____

Glasses of Water: _____

Let's Get Physical: _____
_____
_____
_____

How Am I Doing?: _____
_____
_____
_____

TUESDAY

Date: _____

Total Daily Net Carb Intake: _____

BREAKFAST:

Net Carbs: _____

LUNCH:

Net Carbs: _____

DINNER:

Net Carbs: _____

SNACKS:
  Morning:
  Afternoon:
  Evening:

Net Carbs: _____

Glasses of Water: _____

Let's Get Physical: _____
_____
_____
_____

How Am I Doing?: _____
_____
_____
_____

WEDNESDAY

Date: _____

Total Daily Net Carb Intake: _____

BREAKFAST:

Net Carbs: _____

LUNCH:

Net Carbs: _____

DINNER:

Net Carbs: _____

SNACKS:
  Morning:
  Afternoon:
  Evening:

Net Carbs: _____

Glasses of Water: _____

Let's Get Physical: _____
_____
_____
_____

How Am I Doing?: _____
_____
_____
_____

THURSDAY

Date: _____

Total Daily Net Carb Intake: _____

BREAKFAST:

Net Carbs: _____

LUNCH:

Net Carbs: _____

DINNER:

Net Carbs: _____

SNACKS:
  Morning:
  Afternoon:
  Evening:

Net Carbs: _____

Glasses of Water: _____

Let's Get Physical: _____
_____
_____
_____

How Am I Doing?: _____
_____
_____
_____

FRIDAY

Date: _____

Total Daily Net Carb Intake: _____

BREAKFAST:

Net Carbs: _____

LUNCH:

Net Carbs: _____

DINNER:

Net Carbs: _____

SNACKS:
   Morning:
   Afternoon:
   Evening:

Net Carbs: _____

Glasses of Water: _____

Let's Get Physical: _____

_____

_____

How Am I Doing?: _____

_____

_____

_____

SATURDAY

Date: _____

Total Daily Net Carb Intake: _____

BREAKFAST:

Net Carbs: _____

LUNCH:

Net Carbs: _____

DINNER:

Net Carbs: _____

SNACKS:
  Morning:
  Afternoon:
  Evening:

Net Carbs: _____

Glasses of Water: _____

Let's Get Physical: _____
_____
_____
_____

How Am I Doing?: _____
_____
_____
_____

WEEK SEVENTEEN

Congratulations! You've now completed sixteen weeks of your new low-carb lifestyle. But check your diary—have you been getting physical?

One of the simplest ways to exercise—no pool or gym required—is to pull a pair of sneakers out of your closet and start walking.

- Make a commitment to walk with a regular partner or group at least three or four days a week.
- Set aside specific walking times that you can stick to. (Most people find mornings best.)
- To keep it interesting, vary your walks.
- Don't let foul weather deter you. Equip yourself with a poncho in case of rain, and warm, layered clothing for winter months.

Daily Carb Quota: _____

SUNDAY

Date: _____

Total Daily Net Carb Intake: _____

BREAKFAST:

Net Carbs: _____

LUNCH:

Net Carbs: _____

DINNER:

Net Carbs: _____

SNACKS:
  Morning:
  Afternoon:
  Evening:

Net Carbs: _____

Glasses of Water: _____

Let's Get Physical: _____
_____
_____
_____

How Am I Doing?: _____
_____
_____
_____

MONDAY

Date: _____

Total Daily Net Carb Intake: _____

BREAKFAST:

Net Carbs: _____

LUNCH:

Net Carbs: _____

DINNER:

Net Carbs: _____

SNACKS:
  Morning:
  Afternoon:
  Evening:

Net Carbs: _____

Glasses of Water: _____

Let's Get Physical: _____
_____
_____
_____

How Am I Doing?: _____
_____
_____
_____

TUESDAY

Date: _____

Total Daily Net Carb Intake: _____

BREAKFAST:

Net Carbs: _____

LUNCH:

Net Carbs: _____

DINNER:

Net Carbs: _____

SNACKS:
  Morning:
  Afternoon:
  Evening:

Net Carbs: _____

Glasses of Water: _____

Let's Get Physical: _____
_____
_____
_____

How Am I Doing?: _____
_____
_____
_____

WEDNESDAY

Date: _____

Total Daily Net Carb Intake: _____

BREAKFAST:

Net Carbs: _____

LUNCH:

Net Carbs: _____

DINNER:

Net Carbs: _____

SNACKS:
  Morning:
  Afternoon:
  Evening:

Net Carbs: _____

Glasses of Water: _____

Let's Get Physical: _____
_____
_____
_____

How Am I Doing?: _____
_____
_____
_____

THURSDAY

Date: _____

Total Daily Net Carb Intake: _____

BREAKFAST:

Net Carbs: _____

LUNCH:

Net Carbs: _____

DINNER:

Net Carbs: _____

SNACKS:
  Morning:
  Afternoon:
  Evening:

Net Carbs: _____

Glasses of Water: _____

Let's Get Physical: _____
_____
_____
_____

How Am I Doing?: _____
_____
_____
_____

FRIDAY

Date: _____

Total Daily Net Carb Intake: _____

BREAKFAST:

Net Carbs: _____

LUNCH:

Net Carbs: _____

DINNER:

Net Carbs: _____

SNACKS:
  Morning:
  Afternoon:
  Evening:

Net Carbs: _____

Glasses of Water: _____

Let's Get Physical: _____
_____
_____
_____

How Am I Doing?: _____
_____
_____
_____

SATURDAY

Date: _____

Total Daily Net Carb Intake: _____

BREAKFAST:

Net Carbs: _____

LUNCH:

Net Carbs: _____

DINNER:

Net Carbs: _____

SNACKS:
　　Morning:
　　Afternoon:
　　Evening:

Net Carbs: _____

Glasses of Water: _____

Let's Get Physical: _____
_____
_____
_____

How Am I Doing?: _____
_____
_____
_____

WEEK EIGHTEEN

The incredible, edible egg is back on the menu! Yes, with their high cholesterol count, eggs once suffered from a bad reputation heartwise, but more recent nutritional thinking focuses on saturated fat, refined carbs, and sugar—not dietary cholesterol—as the major culprits in heart disease. Eggs are high in protein and other nutrients and are low in sodium. They're a great way to start the day, and hard-boiled eggs make a healthy snack at any hour. You can also mix hard-boiled eggs with regular or flavored mayonnaise to make a tasty egg salad. (If you add celery for more texture and flavor, be sure to include those additional carbs in your daily net carb count.)

Daily Carb Quota: _____

SUNDAY

Date: _____

Total Daily Net Carb Intake: _____

BREAKFAST:

Net Carbs: _____

LUNCH:

Net Carbs: _____

DINNER:

Net Carbs: _____

SNACKS:
   Morning:
   Afternoon:
   Evening:

Net Carbs: _____

Glasses of Water: _____

Let's Get Physical: _____
_____
_____
_____

How Am I Doing?: _____
_____
_____
_____

MONDAY

Date: _____

Total Daily Net Carb Intake: _____

BREAKFAST:

Net Carbs: _____

LUNCH:

Net Carbs: _____

DINNER:

Net Carbs: _____

SNACKS:
  Morning:
  Afternoon:
  Evening:

Net Carbs: _____

Glasses of Water: _____

Let's Get Physical: _____
_____
_____
_____

How Am I Doing?: _____
_____
_____
_____

TUESDAY

Date: _____

Total Daily Net Carb Intake: _____

BREAKFAST:

Net Carbs: _____

LUNCH:

Net Carbs: _____

DINNER:

Net Carbs: _____

SNACKS:
  Morning:
  Afternoon:
  Evening:

Net Carbs: _____

Glasses of Water: _____

Let's Get Physical: _____
_____
_____
_____

How Am I Doing?: _____
_____
_____
_____

WEDNESDAY

Date: _____

Total Daily Net Carb Intake: _____

BREAKFAST:

Net Carbs: _____

LUNCH:

Net Carbs: _____

DINNER:

Net Carbs: _____

SNACKS:
   Morning:
   Afternoon:
   Evening:

Net Carbs: _____

Glasses of Water: _____

Let's Get Physical: _____
_____
_____
_____

How Am I Doing?: _____
_____
_____
_____

THURSDAY

Date: _____

Total Daily Net Carb Intake: _____

BREAKFAST:

Net Carbs: _____

LUNCH:

Net Carbs: _____

DINNER:

Net Carbs: _____

SNACKS:
  Morning:
  Afternoon:
  Evening:

Net Carbs: _____

Glasses of Water: _____

Let's Get Physical: _____
_____
_____
_____

How Am I Doing?: _____
_____
_____
_____

FRIDAY

Date: _____

Total Daily Net Carb Intake: _____

BREAKFAST:

Net Carbs: _____

LUNCH:

Net Carbs: _____

DINNER:

Net Carbs: _____

SNACKS:
  Morning:
  Afternoon:
  Evening:

Net Carbs: _____

Glasses of Water: _____

Let's Get Physical: _____
_____
_____
_____

How Am I Doing?: _____
_____
_____
_____

SATURDAY

Date: _____

Total Daily Net Carb Intake: _____

BREAKFAST:

Net Carbs: _____

LUNCH:

Net Carbs: _____

DINNER:

Net Carbs: _____

SNACKS:
   Morning:
   Afternoon:
   Evening:

Net Carbs: _____

Glasses of Water: _____

Let's Get Physical: _____
_____
_____
_____

How Am I Doing?: _____
_____
_____
_____

WEEK NINETEEN

Steer clear of trans-fatty acids. Created by adding hydrogen to vegetable oil (which solidifies it and increases shelf life), these are the worst fats. They not only raise the levels of "bad" LDL cholesterol and triglycerides, they also lower the level of "good" HDL cholesterol. The good news is that your low-carb lifestyle is naturally low in trans fats, which are found in highly processed foods such as cookies, crackers, doughnuts, margarine, imitation cheese, French fries, and chicken nuggets. Trans fats are usually listed on food labels as partially hydrogenated oils.

Daily Carb Quota: _____

SUNDAY

Date: _____

Total Daily Net Carb Intake: _____

BREAKFAST:

Net Carbs: _____

LUNCH:

Net Carbs: _____

DINNER:

Net Carbs: _____

SNACKS:
  Morning:
  Afternoon:
  Evening:

Net Carbs: _____

Glasses of Water: _____

Let's Get Physical: _____
_____
_____
_____

How Am I Doing?: _____
_____
_____
_____

MONDAY

Date: _____

Total Daily Net Carb Intake: _____

BREAKFAST:

Net Carbs: _____

LUNCH:

Net Carbs: _____

DINNER:

Net Carbs: _____

SNACKS:
  Morning:
  Afternoon:
  Evening:

Net Carbs: _____

Glasses of Water: _____

Let's Get Physical: _____
_____
_____
_____

How Am I Doing?: _____
_____
_____
_____

TUESDAY

Date: _____

Total Daily Net Carb Intake: _____

BREAKFAST:

Net Carbs: _____

LUNCH:

Net Carbs: _____

DINNER:

Net Carbs: _____

SNACKS:
 Morning:
 Afternoon:
 Evening:

Net Carbs: _____

Glasses of Water: _____

Let's Get Physical: _____
_____
_____
_____

How Am I Doing?: _____
_____
_____
_____

WEDNESDAY

Date: _____

Total Daily Net Carb Intake: _____

BREAKFAST:

Net Carbs: _____

LUNCH:

Net Carbs: _____

DINNER:

Net Carbs: _____

SNACKS:
  Morning:
  Afternoon:
  Evening:

Net Carbs: _____

Glasses of Water: _____

Let's Get Physical: _____
_____
_____
_____

How Am I Doing?: _____
_____
_____
_____

THURSDAY

Date: _____

Total Daily Net Carb Intake: _____

BREAKFAST:

Net Carbs: _____

LUNCH:

Net Carbs: _____

DINNER:

Net Carbs: _____

SNACKS:
   Morning:
   Afternoon:
   Evening:

Net Carbs: _____

Glasses of Water: _____

Let's Get Physical: _____
_____
_____
_____

How Am I Doing?: _____
_____
_____
_____

FRIDAY

Date: _____

Total Daily Net Carb Intake: _____

BREAKFAST:

Net Carbs: _____

LUNCH:

Net Carbs: _____

DINNER:

Net Carbs: _____

SNACKS:
   Morning:
   Afternoon:
   Evening:

Net Carbs: _____

Glasses of Water: _____

Let's Get Physical: _____
_____
_____
_____

How Am I Doing?: _____
_____
_____
_____

SATURDAY

Date: _____

Total Daily Net Carb Intake: _____

BREAKFAST:

Net Carbs: _____

LUNCH:

Net Carbs: _____

DINNER:

Net Carbs: _____

SNACKS:
  Morning:
  Afternoon:
  Evening:

Net Carbs: _____

Glasses of Water: _____

Let's Get Physical: _____
_____
_____
_____

How Am I Doing?: _____
_____
_____
_____

WEEK TWENTY

Read labels! Some products are labeled low carb, and others high protein. But do the math yourself: Look at the total number of carbs and subtract grams of fiber to get net carbs. Although it is a carbohydrate, fiber does not convert to glucose and raise your blood sugar. In fact, fiber slows the entry of glucose into your bloodstream and helps you feel fuller.

Remember that net carbs are the ones that you record in your diary each day.

Daily Carb Quota: _____

SUNDAY

Date: _____

Total Daily Net Carb Intake: _____

BREAKFAST:

Net Carbs: _____

LUNCH:

Net Carbs: _____

DINNER:

Net Carbs: _____

SNACKS:
    Morning:
    Afternoon:
    Evening:

Net Carbs: _____

Glasses of Water: _____

Let's Get Physical: _____
_____
_____
_____

How Am I Doing?: _____
_____
_____
_____

MONDAY

Date: _____

Total Daily Net Carb Intake: _____

BREAKFAST:

Net Carbs: _____

LUNCH:

Net Carbs: _____

DINNER:

Net Carbs: _____

SNACKS:
   Morning:
   Afternoon:
   Evening:

Net Carbs: _____

Glasses of Water: _____

Let's Get Physical: _____
_____
_____
_____

How Am I Doing?: _____
_____
_____
_____

TUESDAY

Date: _____

Total Daily Net Carb Intake: _____

BREAKFAST:

Net Carbs: _____

LUNCH:

Net Carbs: _____

DINNER:

Net Carbs: _____

SNACKS:
   Morning:
   Afternoon:
   Evening:

Net Carbs: _____

Glasses of Water: _____

Let's Get Physical: _____
_____
_____
_____

How Am I Doing?: _____
_____
_____
_____

WEDNESDAY

Date: _____

Total Daily Net Carb Intake: _____

BREAKFAST:

Net Carbs: _____

LUNCH:

Net Carbs: _____

DINNER:

Net Carbs: _____

SNACKS:
   Morning:
   Afternoon:
   Evening:

Net Carbs: _____

Glasses of Water: _____

Let's Get Physical: _____
_____
_____
_____

How Am I Doing?: _____
_____
_____
_____

THURSDAY

Date: _____

Total Daily Net Carb Intake: _____

BREAKFAST:

Net Carbs: _____

LUNCH:

Net Carbs: _____

DINNER:

Net Carbs: _____

SNACKS:
 Morning:
 Afternoon:
 Evening:

Net Carbs: _____

Glasses of Water: _____

Let's Get Physical: _____
_____
_____
_____

How Am I Doing?: _____
_____
_____
_____

FRIDAY

Date: _____

Total Daily Net Carb Intake: _____

BREAKFAST:

Net Carbs: _____

LUNCH:

Net Carbs: _____

DINNER:

Net Carbs: _____

SNACKS:
  Morning:
  Afternoon:
  Evening:

Net Carbs: _____

Glasses of Water: _____

Let's Get Physical: _____

_____

_____

How Am I Doing?: _____

_____

_____

SATURDAY

Date: _____

Total Daily Net Carb Intake: _____

BREAKFAST:

Net Carbs: _____

LUNCH:

Net Carbs: _____

DINNER:

Net Carbs: _____

SNACKS:
  Morning:
  Afternoon:
  Evening:

Net Carbs: _____

Glasses of Water: _____

Let's Get Physical: _____
_____
_____
_____

How Am I Doing?: _____
_____
_____
_____

WEEK TWENTY-ONE

Congratulations! You've completed twenty weeks of your new low-carb lifestyle. Now is a good moment to take a deep breath and think about stress and anxiety—states that send many people straight to the refrigerator in search of comfort food.

What's a better way to cope? Meditation. This age-old technique relieves tension and stress, restores balance, and suffuses the body with energy. Choose from one of these three basic types:

- *Mindfulness meditation* is a moment-to-moment awareness of life going on in and around you. Turn your mind away from worries and focus on the present, such as your breathing.
- *Mantra meditation* involves the repetition of a mantra, or spiritually significant word, phrase, or sound. When you sit with your eyes closed and repeat your mantra, you become more calm and relaxed.
- *Visualization* uses images as a focus of meditation. Set aside your problems for a moment and imagine yourself on a beach, listening to the sound of the waves and feeling the warm sand between your toes.

Daily Carb Quota: _____

SUNDAY

Date: _____

Total Daily Net Carb Intake: _____

BREAKFAST:

Net Carbs: _____

LUNCH:

Net Carbs: _____

DINNER:

Net Carbs: _____

SNACKS:
  Morning:
  Afternoon:
  Evening:

Net Carbs: _____

Glasses of Water: _____

Let's Get Physical: _____

_____
_____
_____

How Am I Doing?: _____

_____
_____
_____

MONDAY

Date: _____

Total Daily Net Carb Intake: _____

BREAKFAST:

Net Carbs: _____

LUNCH:

Net Carbs: _____

DINNER:

Net Carbs: _____

SNACKS:
  Morning:
  Afternoon:
  Evening:

Net Carbs: _____

Glasses of Water: _____

Let's Get Physical: _____

_____

_____

_____

How Am I Doing?: _____

_____

_____

_____

TUESDAY

Date: _____

Total Daily Net Carb Intake: _____

BREAKFAST:

Net Carbs: _____

LUNCH:

Net Carbs: _____

DINNER:

Net Carbs: _____

SNACKS:
   Morning:
   Afternoon:
   Evening:

Net Carbs: _____

Glasses of Water: _____

Let's Get Physical: _____
_____
_____
_____

How Am I Doing?: _____
_____
_____
_____

WEDNESDAY

Date: _____

Total Daily Net Carb Intake: _____

BREAKFAST:

Net Carbs: _____

LUNCH:

Net Carbs: _____

DINNER:

Net Carbs: _____

SNACKS:
  Morning:
  Afternoon:
  Evening:

Net Carbs: _____

Glasses of Water: _____

Let's Get Physical: _____
_____
_____
_____

How Am I Doing?: _____
_____
_____
_____

THURSDAY

Date: _____

Total Daily Net Carb Intake: _____

BREAKFAST:

Net Carbs: _____

LUNCH:

Net Carbs: _____

DINNER:

Net Carbs: _____

SNACKS:
  Morning:
  Afternoon:
  Evening:

Net Carbs: _____

Glasses of Water: _____

Let's Get Physical: _____
_____
_____
_____

How Am I Doing?: _____
_____
_____
_____

FRIDAY

Date: _____

Total Daily Net Carb Intake: _____

BREAKFAST:

Net Carbs: _____

LUNCH:

Net Carbs: _____

DINNER:

Net Carbs: _____

SNACKS:
  Morning:
  Afternoon:
  Evening:

Net Carbs: _____

Glasses of Water: _____

Let's Get Physical: _____
_____
_____
_____

How Am I Doing?: _____
_____
_____
_____

SATURDAY

Date: _____

Total Daily Net Carb Intake: _____

BREAKFAST:

Net Carbs: _____

LUNCH:

Net Carbs: _____

DINNER:

Net Carbs: _____

SNACKS:
    Morning:
    Afternoon:
    Evening:

Net Carbs: _____

Glasses of Water: _____

Let's Get Physical: _____
_____
_____
_____

How Am I Doing?: _____
_____
_____
_____

WEEK TWENTY-TWO

When you snack on yogurt, avoid low-fat products that are packed with carbohydrates. Instead, choose plain whole milk yogurt, sweeten it with a packet of sugar substitute, and add fresh berries.

Daily Carb Quota: _____

SUNDAY

Date: _____

Total Daily Net Carb Intake: _____

BREAKFAST:

Net Carbs: _____

LUNCH:

Net Carbs: _____

DINNER:

Net Carbs: _____

SNACKS:
    Morning:
    Afternoon:
    Evening:

Net Carbs: _____

Glasses of Water: _____

Let's Get Physical: _____
_____
_____
_____

How Am I Doing?: _____
_____
_____
_____

MONDAY

Date: _____

Total Daily Net Carb Intake: _____

BREAKFAST:

Net Carbs: _____

LUNCH:

Net Carbs: _____

DINNER:

Net Carbs: _____

SNACKS:
    Morning:
    Afternoon:
    Evening:

Net Carbs: _____

Glasses of Water: _____

Let's Get Physical: _____
_____
_____
_____

How Am I Doing?: _____
_____
_____
_____

TUESDAY

Date: _____

Total Daily Net Carb Intake: _____

BREAKFAST:

Net Carbs: _____

LUNCH:

Net Carbs: _____

DINNER:

Net Carbs: _____

SNACKS:
   Morning:
   Afternoon:
   Evening:

Net Carbs: _____

Glasses of Water: _____

Let's Get Physical: _____
_____
_____
_____

How Am I Doing?: _____
_____
_____
_____

WEDNESDAY

Date: _____

Total Daily Net Carb Intake: _____

BREAKFAST:

Net Carbs: _____

LUNCH:

Net Carbs: _____

DINNER:

Net Carbs: _____

SNACKS:
  Morning:
  Afternoon:
  Evening:

Net Carbs: _____

Glasses of Water: _____

Let's Get Physical: _____

_____

_____

_____

How Am I Doing?: _____

_____

_____

_____

THURSDAY

Date: _____

Total Daily Net Carb Intake: _____

BREAKFAST:

Net Carbs: _____

LUNCH:

Net Carbs: _____

DINNER:

Net Carbs: _____

SNACKS:
    Morning:
    Afternoon:
    Evening:

Net Carbs: _____

Glasses of Water: _____

Let's Get Physical: _____
_____
_____
_____

How Am I Doing?: _____
_____
_____
_____

FRIDAY

Date: _____

Total Daily Net Carb Intake: _____

BREAKFAST:

Net Carbs: _____

LUNCH:

Net Carbs: _____

DINNER:

Net Carbs: _____

SNACKS:
  Morning:
  Afternoon:
  Evening:

Net Carbs: _____

Glasses of Water: _____

Let's Get Physical: _____
_____
_____
_____

How Am I Doing?: _____
_____
_____
_____

SATURDAY

Date: _____

Total Daily Net Carb Intake: _____

BREAKFAST:

Net Carbs: _____

LUNCH:

Net Carbs: _____

DINNER:

Net Carbs: _____

SNACKS:
    Morning:
    Afternoon:
    Evening:

Net Carbs: _____

Glasses of Water: _____

Let's Get Physical: _____
_____
_____
_____

How Am I Doing?: _____
_____
_____
_____

WEEK TWENTY-THREE

Look for new recipes. Everybody gets tired of the same old foods, no matter what diet plan they are following. To vary your menus, exchange favorite recipes with friends who are also embracing the low-carb lifestyle, and pick up a low-carb cookbook at the library or bookstore. Many recipes are also available online.

Daily Carb Quota: _____

SUNDAY

Date: _____

Total Daily Net Carb Intake: _____

BREAKFAST:

Net Carbs: _____

LUNCH:

Net Carbs: _____

DINNER:

Net Carbs: _____

SNACKS:
    Morning:
    Afternoon:
    Evening:

Net Carbs: _____

Glasses of Water: _____

Let's Get Physical: _____
_____
_____
_____

How Am I Doing?: _____
_____
_____
_____

MONDAY

Date: _____

Total Daily Net Carb Intake: _____

BREAKFAST:

Net Carbs: _____

LUNCH:

Net Carbs: _____

DINNER:

Net Carbs: _____

SNACKS:
   Morning:
   Afternoon:
   Evening:

Net Carbs: _____

Glasses of Water: _____

Let's Get Physical: _____
_____
_____
_____

How Am I Doing?: _____
_____
_____
_____

TUESDAY

Date: _____

Total Daily Net Carb Intake: _____

BREAKFAST:

Net Carbs: _____

LUNCH:

Net Carbs: _____

DINNER:

Net Carbs: _____

SNACKS:
    Morning:
    Afternoon:
    Evening:

Net Carbs: _____

Glasses of Water: _____

Let's Get Physical: _____

_____

_____

_____

How Am I Doing?: _____

_____

_____

_____

WEDNESDAY

Date: _____

Total Daily Net Carb Intake: _____

BREAKFAST:

Net Carbs: _____

LUNCH:

Net Carbs: _____

DINNER:

Net Carbs: _____

SNACKS:
  Morning:
  Afternoon:
  Evening:

Net Carbs: _____

Glasses of Water: _____

Let's Get Physical: _____

_____

_____

_____

How Am I Doing?: _____

_____

_____

_____

THURSDAY

Date: _____

Total Daily Net Carb Intake: _____

BREAKFAST:

Net Carbs: _____

LUNCH:

Net Carbs: _____

DINNER:

Net Carbs: _____

SNACKS:
    Morning:
    Afternoon:
    Evening:

Net Carbs: _____

Glasses of Water: _____

Let's Get Physical: _____
_____
_____
_____

How Am I Doing?: _____
_____
_____

FRIDAY

Date: _____

Total Daily Net Carb Intake: _____

BREAKFAST:

Net Carbs: _____

LUNCH:

Net Carbs: _____

DINNER:

Net Carbs: _____

SNACKS:
  Morning:
  Afternoon:
  Evening:

Net Carbs: _____

Glasses of Water: _____

Let's Get Physical: _____
_____
_____
_____

How Am I Doing?: _____
_____
_____
_____

SATURDAY

Date: _____

Total Daily Net Carb Intake: _____

BREAKFAST:

Net Carbs: _____

LUNCH:

Net Carbs: _____

DINNER:

Net Carbs: _____

SNACKS:
    Morning:
    Afternoon:
    Evening:

Net Carbs: _____

Glasses of Water: _____

Let's Get Physical: _____
_____
_____
_____

How Am I Doing?: _____
_____
_____
_____

WEEK TWENTY-FOUR

Abandon processed bread crumbs and croutons! Sure, we all like texture, but there are healthier ways to achieve this effect. For instance, sprinkle nuts or seeds on salads and vegetables. Or get even more creative: Chop up three pecans, mix with a teaspoon of butter, tuck them under the skin of a chicken breast, and broil. Or mix ground nuts with prepared horseradish and a dash of olive oil to top a salmon steak. You can also make your own bread crumbs and croutons from toasted low-carb bread.

Daily Carb Quota: _____

SUNDAY

Date: _____

Total Daily Net Carb Intake: _____

BREAKFAST:

Net Carbs: _____

LUNCH:

Net Carbs: _____

DINNER:

Net Carbs: _____

SNACKS:
Morning:
Afternoon:
Evening:

Net Carbs: _____

Glasses of Water: _____

Let's Get Physical: _____

_____

_____

_____

How Am I Doing?: _____

_____

_____

_____

MONDAY

Date: _____

Total Daily Net Carb Intake: _____

BREAKFAST:

Net Carbs: _____

LUNCH:

Net Carbs: _____

DINNER:

Net Carbs: _____

SNACKS:
  Morning:
  Afternoon:
  Evening:

Net Carbs: _____

Glasses of Water: _____

Let's Get Physical: _____

_____

_____

_____

How Am I Doing?: _____

_____

_____

_____

TUESDAY

Date: _____

Total Daily Net Carb Intake: _____

BREAKFAST:

Net Carbs: _____

LUNCH:

Net Carbs: _____

DINNER:

Net Carbs: _____

SNACKS:
   Morning:
   Afternoon:
   Evening:

Net Carbs: _____

Glasses of Water: _____

Let's Get Physical: _____
_____
_____
_____

How Am I Doing?: _____
_____
_____
_____

WEDNESDAY

Date: _____

Total Daily Net Carb Intake: _____

BREAKFAST:

Net Carbs: _____

LUNCH:

Net Carbs: _____

DINNER:

Net Carbs: _____

SNACKS:
   Morning:
   Afternoon:
   Evening:

Net Carbs: _____

Glasses of Water: _____

Let's Get Physical: _____
_____
_____
_____

How Am I Doing?: _____
_____
_____
_____

THURSDAY

Date: _____

Total Daily Net Carb Intake: _____

BREAKFAST:

Net Carbs: _____

LUNCH:

Net Carbs: _____

DINNER:

Net Carbs: _____

SNACKS:
 Morning:
 Afternoon:
 Evening:

Net Carbs: _____

Glasses of Water: _____

Let's Get Physical: _____
_____
_____
_____

How Am I Doing?: _____
_____
_____
_____

FRIDAY

Date: _____

Total Daily Net Carb Intake: _____

BREAKFAST:

Net Carbs: _____

LUNCH:

Net Carbs: _____

DINNER:

Net Carbs: _____

SNACKS:
  Morning:
  Afternoon:
  Evening:

Net Carbs: _____

Glasses of Water: _____

Let's Get Physical: _____
_____
_____
_____

How Am I Doing?: _____
_____
_____
_____

SATURDAY

Date: _____

Total Daily Net Carb Intake: _____

BREAKFAST:

Net Carbs: _____

LUNCH:

Net Carbs: _____

DINNER:

Net Carbs: _____

SNACKS:
Morning:
Afternoon:
Evening:

Net Carbs: _____

Glasses of Water: _____

Let's Get Physical: _____
_____
_____
_____

How Am I Doing?: _____
_____
_____
_____

WEEK TWENTY-FIVE

The more exercise you get, the more carbs you can consume without putting on weight. Now that you've been working out regularly for several months, think about fine-tuning your exercise program—maybe even investing in a few sessions with a personal trainer.

The best regimens include a combination of three forms of exercise:

- Aerobic, including brisk walks or biking
- Resistance training, such as using free weights
- Stretching to increase flexibility

Daily Carb Quota: _____

SUNDAY

Date: _____

Total Daily Net Carb Intake: _____

BREAKFAST:

Net Carbs: _____

LUNCH:

Net Carbs: _____

DINNER:

Net Carbs: _____

SNACKS:
  Morning:
  Afternoon:
  Evening:

Net Carbs: _____

Glasses of Water: _____

Let's Get Physical: _____
_____
_____
_____

How Am I Doing?: _____
_____
_____
_____

MONDAY

Date: _____

Total Daily Net Carb Intake: _____

BREAKFAST:

Net Carbs: _____

LUNCH:

Net Carbs: _____

DINNER:

Net Carbs: _____

SNACKS:
  Morning:
  Afternoon:
  Evening:

Net Carbs: _____

Glasses of Water: _____

Let's Get Physical: _____
_____
_____
_____

How Am I Doing?: _____
_____
_____
_____

TUESDAY

Date: _____

Total Daily Net Carb Intake: _____

BREAKFAST:

Net Carbs: _____

LUNCH:

Net Carbs: _____

DINNER:

Net Carbs: _____

SNACKS:
  Morning:
  Afternoon:
  Evening:

Net Carbs: _____

Glasses of Water: _____

Let's Get Physical: _____
_____
_____
_____

How Am I Doing?: _____
_____
_____
_____

WEDNESDAY

Date: _____

Total Daily Net Carb Intake: _____

BREAKFAST:

Net Carbs: _____

LUNCH:

Net Carbs: _____

DINNER:

Net Carbs: _____

SNACKS:
   Morning:
   Afternoon:
   Evening:

Net Carbs: _____

Glasses of Water: _____

Let's Get Physical: _____
_____
_____
_____

How Am I Doing?: _____
_____
_____
_____

THURSDAY

Date: _____

Total Daily Net Carb Intake: _____

BREAKFAST:

Net Carbs: _____

LUNCH:

Net Carbs: _____

DINNER:

Net Carbs: _____

SNACKS:
  Morning:
  Afternoon:
  Evening:

Net Carbs: _____

Glasses of Water: _____

Let's Get Physical: _____
_____
_____
_____

How Am I Doing?: _____
_____
_____
_____

FRIDAY

Date: _____

Total Daily Net Carb Intake: _____

BREAKFAST:

Net Carbs: _____

LUNCH:

Net Carbs: _____

DINNER:

Net Carbs: _____

SNACKS:
  Morning:
  Afternoon:
  Evening:

Net Carbs: _____

Glasses of Water: _____

Let's Get Physical: _____
_____
_____
_____

How Am I Doing?: _____
_____
_____
_____

SATURDAY

Date: _____

Total Daily Net Carb Intake: _____

BREAKFAST:

Net Carbs: _____

LUNCH:

Net Carbs: _____

DINNER:

Net Carbs: _____

SNACKS:
  Morning:
  Afternoon:
  Evening:

Net Carbs: _____

Glasses of Water: _____

Let's Get Physical: _____
_____
_____
_____

How Am I Doing?: _____
_____
_____
_____

WEEK TWENTY-SIX

Congratulations! You've made it to the final week! Take this moment to celebrate the weight you've lost. Whether it's five pounds or twenty-five pounds, you've come a long way in your twenty-six-week journey. Eating low-carb foods is no longer a diet for you—it's a healthy way of life. You look better, feel better, and weigh less, and chances are, when you visit your doctor, you'll find that your cholesterol, triglyceride, and blood sugar levels are a positive reflection of your new low-carb lifestyle. But just because you've come to the end of your journal, don't think of this as an end—it's only the beginning of your healthy new life!

To see how far you've come, record your stats.

Starting Weight:	_____
Weight at Halfway Mark:	_____
Current Weight:	_____
Target Weight:	_____
Starting Clothing Size:	_____
Clothing Size at Halfway Mark:	_____
Current Clothing Size:	_____
Target Clothing Size:	_____
Starting Waist Measurement:	_____
Waist Measurement at Halfway Mark:	_____
Current Waist Measurement:	_____
Target Waist Measurement:	_____
Daily Carb Quota:	_____

SUNDAY

Date: _____

Total Daily Net Carb Intake: _____

BREAKFAST:

Net Carbs: _____

LUNCH:

Net Carbs: _____

DINNER:

Net Carbs: _____

SNACKS:
   Morning:
   Afternoon:
   Evening:

Net Carbs: _____

Glasses of Water: _____

Let's Get Physical: _____
_____
_____
_____

How Am I Doing?: _____
_____
_____
_____

MONDAY

Date: _____

Total Daily Net Carb Intake: _____

BREAKFAST:

Net Carbs: _____

LUNCH:

Net Carbs: _____

DINNER:

Net Carbs: _____

SNACKS:
   Morning:
   Afternoon:
   Evening:

Net Carbs: _____

Glasses of Water: _____

Let's Get Physical: _____

_____

_____

_____

How Am I Doing?: _____

_____

_____

_____

TUESDAY

Date: _____

Total Daily Net Carb Intake: _____

BREAKFAST:

Net Carbs: _____

LUNCH:

Net Carbs: _____

DINNER:

Net Carbs: _____

SNACKS:
   Morning:
   Afternoon:
   Evening:

Net Carbs: _____

Glasses of Water: _____

Let's Get Physical: _____
_____
_____
_____

How Am I Doing?: _____
_____
_____
_____

WEDNESDAY

Date: _____

Total Daily Net Carb Intake: _____

BREAKFAST:

Net Carbs: _____

LUNCH:

Net Carbs: _____

DINNER:

Net Carbs: _____

SNACKS:
  Morning:
  Afternoon:
  Evening:

Net Carbs: _____

Glasses of Water: _____

Let's Get Physical: _____
_____
_____
_____

How Am I Doing?: _____
_____
_____
_____

THURSDAY

Date: _____

Total Daily Net Carb Intake: _____

BREAKFAST:

Net Carbs: _____

LUNCH:

Net Carbs: _____

DINNER:

Net Carbs: _____

SNACKS:
  Morning:
  Afternoon:
  Evening:

Net Carbs: _____

Glasses of Water: _____

Let's Get Physical: _____
_____
_____
_____

How Am I Doing?: _____
_____
_____
_____

FRIDAY

Date: _____

Total Daily Net Carb Intake: _____

BREAKFAST:

Net Carbs: _____

LUNCH:

Net Carbs: _____

DINNER:

Net Carbs: _____

SNACKS:
  Morning:
  Afternoon:
  Evening:

Net Carbs: _____

Glasses of Water: _____

Let's Get Physical: _____
_____
_____
_____

How Am I Doing?: _____
_____
_____
_____

SATURDAY

Date: _____

Total Daily Net Carb Intake: _____

BREAKFAST:

Net Carbs: _____

LUNCH:

Net Carbs: _____

DINNER:

Net Carbs: _____

SNACKS:
  Morning:
  Afternoon:
  Evening:

Net Carbs: _____

Glasses of Water: _____

Let's Get Physical: _____
_____
_____
_____

How Am I Doing?: _____
_____
_____
_____

Carbohydrate Gram Counter

FOOD and AMOUNT	CARBS (Grams)	FIBER (Grams)	NET CARBS (Grams)	CALORIES
Baked Goods and Snacks				
Bagel, plain (3½" diameter)	37.9	1.6	36.3	195
Biscuit (2½" diameter)	26.8	0.9	25.9	212
Brownie (1)	27	1	26	190
Cake, angel food (1 slice)	29.2	0.1	29.1	128
Cake, chocolate layer (1 slice)	38	2	36	270
Cookie, chocolate chip (2)	11.3	0	11.3	87
Cookie, oatmeal (2)	33.4	1.5	31.9	212
Cookie, shortbread (2)	10.3	0.3	10	80
Corn chips (20)	9.4	0.6	8.8	100
Crackers, butter (4)	10	0	10	70
Croissant (1)	27	0	27	170
Danish (1)	32	1	31	300
Doughnut, glazed (1)	26.6	0.7	25.9	242
Italian bread (1 slice)	14.2	0.8	13.4	77
Muffin, blueberry (1)	27.2	1.5	25.7	157
Muffin, bran (1)	23.7	4	19.7	163
Muffin, English (1)	26.2	1.5	24.7	134
Pancake (1)	31.8	1.3	30.5	167
Pie, apple (⅛ pie)	42.5	2	40.5	296
Pie, pecan (1 slice)	67	2	65	550
Pita bread, white (6½" diameter)	33.4	1.3	32.1	165
Pita bread, whole wheat (6½" diameter)	35.2	4.7	30.5	170
Popcorn (1 cup)	5	2	3	35
Potato chips (20)	15	1	14	150
Pretzels (5 twisted)	23.8	1	22.8	114
Raisin bread (1 slice)	14.8	1.2	13.6	78
Roll, white (1 oz)	14.9	0.7	14.2	83
Roll, whole wheat (1 oz)	14.5	2.1	12.4	75
Rye bread (1 slice)	13.7	1.6	12.1	73
Tortilla, corn (1)	12.1	1.4	10.7	58
Tortilla, flour (1)	27.2	1.6	25.6	159
Tortilla chips (20)	22.6	2.3	20.3	180
Waffle (1)	15	0	15	110

Carbohydrate Gram Counter

FOOD and AMOUNT	CARBS (Grams)	FIBER (Grams)	NET CARBS (Grams)	CALORIES
Baked Goods and Snacks (continued)				
White bread (1 slice)	14	0.7	13.3	76
Whole grain bread (1 slice)	13.4	1.2	12.2	74
Beans, Legumes, and Tofu				
Black beans (½ cup)	20.4	7.5	12.9	114
Chickpeas (½ cup)	20	7	13	120
Kidney beans (½ cup)	19.8	8.2	11.6	110
Lentils (½ cup)	19.9	7.8	12.1	115
Lima beans (½ cup)	21.2	7	14.2	115
Pinto beans (½ cup)	21.9	7.4	14.5	117
Refried beans (½ cup)	19.6	6.7	12.9	118
Soybeans (½ cup)	10	3.8	6.2	127
Split peas (½ cup)	20.7	8.1	12.6	116
Tofu, firm (½ cup)	5.4	2.9	2.5	183
Tofu, regular (½ cup)	2.3	0.4	1.9	94
Beef, Veal, and Lamb				
Beef tenderloin (6 oz)	0	0	0	619
Brisket (6 oz)	0	0	0	563
Calves' liver (6 oz)	10.4	0	10.4	304
Corned beef (6 oz)	0.3	0	0.3	449
Eye round (6 oz)	0	0	0	410
Ground chuck (6 oz)	0	0	0	562
Ground round (6 oz)	0	0	0	454
Lamb chop	0	0	0	614
Prime rib (6 oz)	0	0	0	667
Roast beef (6 oz)	0	0	0	576
Shell steak (6 oz)	0	0	0	352
Sirloin steak (6 oz)	0	0	0	344
Skirt steak (6 oz)	0	0	0	568
Veal cutlet (6 oz)	0	0	0	483

Carbohydrate Gram Counter

FOOD and AMOUNT	CARBS (Grams)	FIBER (Grams)	NET CARBS (Grams)	CALORIES
Beverages, Alcoholic				
Beer (12 oz)	13.2	0.7	12.5	146
Beer, light (12 oz)	4.6	0	4.6	99
Liquor (1 oz)	0	0	0	82
Wine, red (3½ oz)	1.8	0	1.8	74
Wine, white (3½ oz)	0.8	0	0.8	70
Beverages, Nonalcoholic				
Apple juice (4 oz)	14.5	0.1	14.4	58
Carrot juice (4 oz)	5.8	0	5.8	25
Coffee (8 oz)	1	0	1	5
Cola (12 oz)	38.7	0	38.7	153
Cranberry juice (4 oz)	18.2	0.1	18.1	72
Diet soda (12 oz)	0	0	0	0
Ginger ale (12 oz)	31.8	0	31.8	124
Grape juice (4 oz)	18.9	0.1	18.8	77
Orange juice (4 oz)	12.9	0.3	12.6	56
Prune juice (4 oz)	22.3	1.3	21	91
Seltzer/club soda (12 oz)	0	0	0	0
Tea (8 oz)	0.7	0	0.7	2
Tomato juice (4 oz)	5.1	1	4.1	21
Cheese				
American (1 slice)	0.3	0	0.3	79
Brie (1 oz)	0.1	0	0.1	95
Camembert (1 oz)	0.1	0	0.1	85
Cheddar (1 oz)	0.4	0	0.4	114
Cottage (½ cup)	4.1	0	4.1	101
Gorgonzola (1 oz)	0	0	0	111
Gouda (1 oz)	0.6	0	0.6	101
Jarlsberg (1 oz)	1	0	1	107
Mozzarella, part skim (1 oz)	0.8	0	0.8	72
Mozzarella, whole milk (1 oz)	0.6	0	0.6	80
Muenster (1 oz)	0.3	0	0.3	104
Parmesan, grated (1 tbsp)	0.2	0	0.2	28
Provolone (1 oz)	0.6	0	0.6	100
Ricotta, part skim (¼ cup)	3.2	0	3.2	85

Carbohydrate Gram Counter

FOOD and AMOUNT	CARBS (Grams)	FIBER (Grams)	NET CARBS (Grams)	CALORIES
Cheese (continued)				
Ricotta, whole milk (¼ cup)	1.9	0	1.9	107
Romano, grated (1 tbsp)	0.2	0	0.2	24
Swiss (1 oz)	1	0	1	107
Condiments, Oils, Seasonings, and Sauces				
Barbecue sauce (1 tbsp)	6	0	6	25
Catsup/ketchup (1 tbsp)	4.2	0.2	4	16
Chocolate syrup (1 tbsp)	11.9	0.5	11.4	51
Cocktail sauce (2 tbsp)	6.5	0.2	6.3	30
Corn syrup (1 tbsp)	15.7	0	15.7	58
Ginger root (1 tbsp)	0.9	0.1	0.8	4
Gravy (2 tbsp)	1.4	0.1	1.3	15
Herbs, dried (1 tsp)	1	0.6	0.4	5
Honey (1 tsp)	5.8	0	5.8	21
Jam/preserves (1 tsp)	4.6	0.1	4.5	19
Jelly, grape (1 tbsp)	4.7	0	4.7	20
Maple syrup (1 tbsp)	13.4	0	13.4	52
Margarine, hard (1 tbsp)	0.1	0	0.1	101
Margarine, soft (1 tbsp)	0.1	0	0.1	102
Mayonnaise (1 tbsp)	0.1	0	0.1	100
Molasses (1 tsp)	4.4	0	4.4	17
Mustard (1 tsp)	0.4	0.2	0.2	3
Oil, canola (1 tbsp)	0	0	0	124
Oil, corn (1 tbsp)	0	0	0	120
Oil, olive (1 tbsp)	0	0	0	119
Oil, peanut (1 tbsp)	0	0	0	119
Olives, green (5)	0.3	0.2	0.1	23
Pesto (2 tbsp)	2	0.9	1.1	155
Salad dressing, balsamic vinaigrette (2 tbsp)	3	0	3	100
Salad dressing, blue cheese (2 tbsp)	2	0	2	170
Salad dressing, French (2 tbsp)	5	0	5	120
Salad dressing, honey Dijon (2 tbsp)	9	0	9	130

Carbohydrate Gram Counter

FOOD and AMOUNT	CARBS (Grams)	FIBER (Grams)	NET CARBS (Grams)	CALORIES
Condiments, Oils, Seasonings, and Sauces (continued)				
Salad dressing, Italian (2 tbsp)	3	0	3	100
Salad dressing, Russian (2 tbsp)	15	0	15	110
Salsa (2 tbsp)	2	0.5	1.5	9
Soy sauce (1 tbsp)	1.5	0	1.5	10
Steak sauce (1 tbsp)	2.4	0.3	2.1	9
Sugar, brown (1 tsp)	4.5	0	4.5	17
Sugar, white (1 tsp)	4.2	0	4.2	16
Sugar substitute (1 tbsp)	1.6	0	1.6	6
Tomato sauce (¼ cup)	4.4	0.9	3.5	18
Vinegar, balsamic (1 tbsp)	2.3	0	2.3	10
Vinegar, cider (1 tbsp)	0.9	0	0.9	2
Vinegar, red (1 tbsp)	1.5	0	1.5	5
Vinegar, rice (1 tbsp)	0	0	0	0
Vinegar, white (1 tbsp)	0	0	0	5
Eggs				
Fried (1)	0.6	0	0.6	92
Poached or boiled (1)	0.6	0	0.6	78
Fish and Seafood				
Anchovies (1)	0	0	0	8
Bass (6 oz)	0	0	0	211
Clams (6 oz)	8.7	0	8.7	252
Cod (6 oz)	0	0	0	179
Crab (6 oz)	0	0	0	168
Haddock (6 oz)	0	0	0	187
Halibut (6 oz)	0	0	0	238
Herring (¼ cup)	8	0	8	120
Lobster (6 oz)	2.2	0	2.2	167
Mackerel (6 oz)	0	0	0	446
Mahimahi (6 oz)	0	0	0	193
Mussels (6 oz)	12.6	0	12.6	293
Oysters (6 oz)	6.7	0	6.7	117

Carbohydrate Gram Counter

FOOD and AMOUNT	CARBS (Grams)	FIBER (Grams)	NET CARBS (Grams)	CALORIES
Fish and Seafood (continued)				
Salmon (6 oz)	0	0	0	350
Sardines, canned in oil (6 oz)	0	0	0	354
Scallops (6 oz)	4.9	0	4.9	228
Shrimp (6 oz)	0	0	0	168
Swordfish (6 oz)	0	0	0	264
Trout (6 oz)	0	0	0	323
Tuna (6 oz)	0	0	0	313
Fruit				
Apple (1)	21	3.8	17.2	82
Apricots (3)	11.7	2.5	9.2	50
Apricots, dried (6 halves)	13	1.9	11.1	50
Avocado, California (½)	6	4.2	1.8	153
Blackberries (½ cup)	9.2	3.8	5.4	37
Blueberries (½ cup)	10.2	2	8.2	31
Boysenberries (½ cup)	9.2	3.8	5.4	26
Cantaloupe (½ cup)	7.4	0.7	6.7	37
Cherries (½ cup)	6.3	0.8	5.5	57
Grapefruit (½ cup)	9.5	1.7	7.8	31
Grapes, green (½ cup)	14.2	0.8	13.4	30
Grapes, red (½ cup)	7.9	0.5	7.4	31
Honeydew melon (½ cup)	7.8	0.5	7.3	30
Mango (½ cup)	14	1.5	12.5	54
Nectarine (1)	16	2.2	13.8	67
Orange (1)	16.3	3.4	12.9	64
Peach (1)	8.8	1.6	7.2	34
Pear (1)	25.1	4	21.1	98
Pineapple (½ cup)	9.6	0.9	8.7	38
Plum (1)	3.7	0.4	3.3	16
Raisins (1 tbsp)	8.1	0.7	7.4	31
Raspberries (½ cup)	7.1	4.2	2.9	30
Strawberries (½ cup)	5.1	1.7	3.4	22
Watermelon (½ cup)	5.5	0.4	5.1	25

Carbohydrate Gram Counter

FOOD and AMOUNT	CARBS (Grams)	FIBER (Grams)	NET CARBS (Grams)	CALORIES
Grains, Cereal, Pasta, and Rice				
Barley (½ cup)	22.2	3	19.2	97
Bran flakes (½ cup)	15.4	3.1	12.3	63
Bulgur (½ cup)	16.9	4.1	12.8	76
Corn flakes (½ cup)	12.1	0.4	11.7	51
Couscous (½ cup)	18.2	1.1	17.1	88
Granola cereal bar (1)	16	2	14	80
Noodles, egg (½ cup)	19.9	0.9	19	106
Oatmeal (½ cup)	12.6	2	10.6	73
Pasta/spaghetti (½ cup)	19.8	0.9	18.9	99
Puffed rice cereal (½ cup)	6.3	0.1	6.2	28
Puffed wheat cereal (½ cup)	10	1	9	45
Rice, brown (½ cup)	22.4	1.8	20.6	108
Rice, white (½ cup)	22.3	0.3	21.9	103
Wheat germ (2 tbsp)	7	1.8	5.2	54
Luncheon Meats and Sausage				
Bologna, beef (3 slices)	2	0	2	266
Bologna, beef and pork (3 slices)	2.4	0	2.4	269
Breakfast sausage (1 link)	1.2	0.7	0.5	32
Frankfurter, beef (1)	1.2	0	1.2	143
Frankfurter, beef and pork (1)	1.5	0	1.5	188
Liverwurst (3 slices)	3.2	1	2.2	176
Olive loaf (3 slices)	7.8	0	7.8	200
Pepperoni (5 pieces)	0.8	0	0.8	137
Salami, beef (3 slices)	1.9	0	1.9	181
Milk, Cream, Butter, Yogurt, and Frozen Desserts				
Butter (1 tbsp)	0	0	0	102
Buttermilk, 1% lowfat (1 cup)	13	0	13	110
Cream, half and half (1 tbsp)	0.5	0	0.5	20
Cream, heavy (1 tbsp)	0.4	0	0.4	51
Cream, light (1 tbsp)	0.6	0	0.6	29
Frozen desserts, non-dairy (½ cup)	21	0	21	200
Ice cream, vanilla (½ cup)	15	0	15	150

Carbohydrate Gram Counter

FOOD and AMOUNT	CARBS (Grams)	FIBER (Grams)	NET CARBS (Grams)	CALORIES
Milk, Cream, Butter, Yogurt, and Frozen Desserts (continued)				
Milk, 1% lowfat (1 cup)	11.7	0	11.7	102
Milk, 2% lowfat (1 cup)	11.7	0	11.7	121
Milk, skim (1 cup)	11.9	0	11.9	86
Milk, whole (1 cup)	11.4	0	11.4	150
Sorbet (½ cup)	30.1	0	30.1	137
Sour cream (2 tbsp)	1.2	0	1.2	62
Soy milk, plain (1 cup)	4.4	3.2	1.2	81
Yogurt, whole (1 cup)	11	0	11	150
Yogurt, frozen vanilla (½ cup)	29	0	29	140
Nuts, Nut Butter, and Seeds				
Almond butter (2 tbsp)	6.8	1.2	5.6	203
Cashews, roasted (2 tbsp)	5.6	0.5	5.1	98
Hazelnuts, roasted (2 tbsp)	2.8	1.6	1.2	106
Peanuts, roasted (2 tbsp)	3.4	1.7	1.7	105
Peanut butter (2 tbsp)	6.9	2.1	4.8	187
Pecans, roasted (2 tbsp)	1.9	1.3	0.6	93
Pistachios (2 tbsp)	4.7	1.6	3.1	88
Pumpkin seeds, hulled (2 tbsp)	4.3	0.3	4	36
Sesame seeds (2 tbsp)	4.2	2.1	2.1	103
Soybeans, roasted (2 tbsp)	7	1.7	5.3	97
Walnuts (2 tbsp)	1.7	0.8	0.9	82
Pork				
Bacon (3 pieces)	0.1	0	0.1	109
Canadian bacon (3 pieces)	0.9	0	0.9	129
Ham (6 oz)	0	0	0	303
Pork chop (6 oz)	0	0	0	344
Ground pork (6 oz)	0	0	0	505
Pork sausage (1)	0.9	0	0.9	183
Prosciutto (6 oz)	0.9	0	0.9	281
Spareribs (6 oz)	0	0	0	675

Carbohydrate Gram Counter

FOOD and AMOUNT	CARBS (Grams)	FIBER (Grams)	NET CARBS (Grams)	CALORIES
Poultry				
Chicken breast (6 oz)	0	0	0	335
Chicken drumstick (6 oz)	0	0	0	367
Chicken leg (6 oz)	0	0	0	379
Chicken thigh (6 oz)	0	0	0	420
Ground turkey (6 oz)	0	0	0	400
Turkey breast (6 oz)	0	0	0	230
Soup				
Beef broth (1 cup)	1	0	1	16
Black bean soup (1 cup)	36	12	24	170
Chicken broth (1 cup)	2	0	2	30
Chicken noodle soup (1 cup)	8.7	0.8	7.9	64
Clam chowder, New England (1 cup)	13	1	2	90
Tomato soup (1 cup)	18	2	16	80
Vegetable soup (1 cup)	16	2	14	90
Vegetables				
Alfalfa sprouts (½ cup)	0.6	0.4	0.2	5
Artichoke (1)	13.4	6.5	6.9	60
Asparagus, steamed (4)	2.5	1	1.5	14
Broccoli (½ cup)	4.9	2.8	2.1	26
Brussel sprouts (½ cup)	6.8	2	4.8	30
Cabbage, green (½ cup)	3.3	1.7	1.6	17
Carrots (½ cup)	8.2	2.6	5.6	35
Cauliflower (½ cup)	2.6	1.7	0.9	14
Celery (1 stalk)	1.5	0.7	0.8	6
Corn (½ cup)	14.7	2.1	12.6	66
Cucumber (½ cup)	1.4	0.4	1	7
Dandelion greens (½ cup)	3.4	1.5	1.9	17
Eggplant (½ cup)	3.3	1.2	2.1	14
Endive (½ cup)	1.8	1.4	0.4	8
Fava beans (½ cup)	16.7	4.6	12.1	94
Fennel (½ cup)	2.8	1.3	1.5	12
Garlic clove (1)	1	0.1	0.9	4
Green beans (½ cup)	4.9	2	2.9	22

Carbohydrate Gram Counter

FOOD and AMOUNT	CARBS (Grams)	FIBER (Grams)	NET CARBS (Grams)	CALORIES
Vegetables (continued)				
Kale (½ cup)	3.4	1.3	2.1	20
Lettuce, Boston (½ cup)	0.7	0.3	0.4	4
Lettuce, iceberg (½ cup)	0.6	0.4	0.2	3
Lettuce, mesclun (½ cup)	1	0.5	0.5	5
Lettuce, romaine (½ cup)	0.7	0.5	0.2	4
Mushrooms (½ cup)	10.4	1.5	8.9	40
Mushroom, Portabello (4 oz)	5.8	1.7	4.1	29
Mustard greens (½ cup)	1.5	1.4	0.1	11
Okra (½ cup)	5.8	2	3.8	26
Onions (½ cup)	6.9	1.4	5.5	30
Parsley (1 tbsp)	0.2	0.1	0.1	1
Parsnips (½ cup)	15.2	3.1	12.1	63
Peas (½ cup)	9.9	3.4	6.5	55
Pepper, green (½ cup)	4.8	1.3	3.5	20
Pepper, red (½ cup)	4.8	1.5	3.3	20
Potatoes (½ cup)	15.6	1.4	14.2	67
Radicchio (½ cup)	0.9	0.2	0.7	5
Radishes (10)	1.6	0.7	0.9	9
Rutabaga (½ cup)	7.4	1.5	5.9	33
Scallions (½ cup)	3.7	1.3	2.4	16
Snow peas (½ cup)	5.6	2.2	3.4	34
Spinach (½ cup)	5.1	2.9	2.2	27
Squash, yellow (½ cup)	3.9	1.3	2.6	18
Sweet potato (½)	13.8	1.7	12.1	59
Tomato, cherry (10)	7.9	1.9	6	36
Tomato, plum (1)	2.9	0.7	2.2	13
Turnip greens (½ cup)	3.1	2.5	0.6	14
Turnips (½ cup)	5.6	2.3	3.3	24
Watercress (½ cup)	0.2	0.2	0	2
Yams (½ cup)	29.7	2.2	27.5	129